YOU CAN'T BEAT ME

YOU CAN'T BEAT ME

DEFYING THE ODDS

Zack Condick

First published in 2024 by Dean Publishing
PO Box 119
Mt. Macedon, Victoria, 3441
Australia
deanpublishing.com

**DEAN
PUBLISHING**

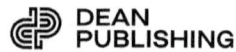

Cataloguing-in-Publication Data
National Library of Australia
Title: You Can't Beat Me
ISBN: 978-1-925452-89-1

Category: Personal health/memoir/healing

Dedication

I dedicate my book to my family, friends, and my beautiful son, who have all supported me through everything, who picked me up when I was down and encouraged me to keep fighting. I wouldn't be here today to tell my story and write this book without you guys.

CONTENTS

A Moment of Devastation

As I sat in emergency, waiting for the results of a leg X-ray, all I wanted was for nothing to be wrong. I just wanted them to fix my broken nose so I could go home and get back to healing my leg.

After what seemed like hours, the doctor came in with the results. "No major breaks," he said. *Phew.* "Just two broken screws."

"Pardon?"

"Just two broken screws."

"Those screws… are holding my leg together."

"Oh, well, they should be able to take them out and put new ones in." I don't think he understood the gravity of the situation. "You should go and see your surgeon."

At that point, there was nothing more the emergency department could do, so, in a panic, I grabbed whatever set of crutches I could find, as I didn't want to put any weight on my bad leg and risk snapping it in half. Then I got in my car and drove myself home.

I called my mate Keiran, crying. I could hardly speak. I was that upset.

"What's wrong?" he asked. "Are you okay? What happened at the hospital?"

"My leg... it's broken. I don't know how I'm going to tell Tessa." We spoke for a bit before ending the call. There was nothing anyone could have said to help the situation.

How do I tell Tessa that, after we've been fighting to save my leg for so long, some drunken idiots might have ruined it all? How do I tell her that everything we've done, everything we've been through might have been for nothing? How do I tell her I could lose my leg?

"

Limits,
like fears,
are often just
an illusion.

– MICHAEL JORDAN

Chapter 1

MY CALLING IN LIFE... OR SO I THOUGHT

Playing with the Big Boys

From a young age, I knew what I wanted to do in life. I wanted to play sport at a high level, and I wanted to be a carpenter, just like my dad.

The first sport I really got into was soccer, which I started playing at around age 5. Naturally, my grandad, being English, was really into soccer, and he may have pushed me into it – not that I needed much pushing. I loved the game and the challenge of competing against the older kids. At the time, the lowest age group in soccer was under sevens, but I didn't let that stop me from joining my older brother Jake's team and playing with the bigger boys. Playing with older kids forced me to push myself. I couldn't just sit in second gear, cruising along, and expect to do well. I was the underdog, and I had to work hard every second I was on the field. But what I lacked in age and experience, I made up for in determination and spirit. Looking back, I was a fighter from the start, always willing to take on whatever came my way. I never backed down from a challenge.

Because I couldn't rely on superior speed, size, or strength, I was forced to develop my skills, which was a blessing. I learnt quickly and was great at adapting to new and challenging situations, many of which I'd face later in life. During those years, fighting to hold my own against the bigger kids, I built a lot of resilience, which was exactly what I needed for what was to come.

When I officially grew into the under-sevens age group, I already had a lot of experience on the field playing against tougher teams and bigger opponents, and suddenly the challenge was gone, so I moved to the Frankston Strikers to play in a more competitive league. During my time with the Strikers, we finished on the top of the ladder several times, and I'd often win the golden boot as the leading goal kicker. I even did training with the Victorian Academy for a couple of years. To anyone watching, it looked like I was well on track to achieve big things in the sport. It looked like I'd found my calling. Then high school happened.

In high school, a lot of my mates were into footy (Aussie rules). It's common for kids to start with soccer when they're young and transition to footy, but probably not so common for someone who was doing so well in the sport. At the time, playing sport with my mates was more important than the sport itself, so I switched to footy and learnt a whole new skill set. With that said, foot skills and coordination do translate to both sports, so I wasn't starting completely from scratch.

Looking back, part of me wishes I'd stuck with soccer to see how far I could've gone with it. In the end, however, footy became my game.

A Jack-of-All-Sports

At age 12, I began my footy career in the under 13s. Surprisingly, the game came naturally to me. I already had the kicking skills and hand-eye coordination, and I knew how to read the play, so the transition was fairly smooth.

Honestly, though, our team wasn't great. We frequently got flogged. But do you know what? It didn't matter, because I loved the game, especially the physical contact, something soccer generally lacks. I should confess – I wasn't playing solely out of a love for the sport or even to play with my mates. Jake and Dad were also into footy and had both won under 18s best and fairests. Part of me was trying to impress them while keeping the family legacy alive, which, for the most part, I did, eventually winning my own under 18s best and fairest award.

I also played cricket from under 13s to under 17s, and I was surprisingly good at that too. Once again, I took to it naturally, playing as an all-rounder. Bat or ball – it didn't matter. I even played Country Week – a competition where the best local kids compete against one another in teams – a couple of years in a row. Even though I was good at cricket and enjoyed the game, I didn't continue through to seniors. At that level, you're playing 80 overs a game, which takes up an entire day. I wasn't keen on the idea. I decided I'd rather spend more time fishing, camping, and motorbike riding.

To me, an entire Saturday of cricket in the scorching sun wasn't appealing in the least when I could be doing other things. Without the drive to succeed in the sport, my focus was better spent elsewhere.

As I got older, still playing footy, I realised that my natural talent would only get me so far. When we're young, we can jump into a sport or any other activity and, if the natural talent is there, do quite well without much effort. However, once we move into higher age brackets, training becomes critical. At a certain point, if we don't actively work to improve our skills, fitness, whatever it might be, the people who work harder quickly overtake us. Knowing this, I put all my effort into footy, aiming high and dreaming big. I knew, if I put in the work, I could achieve great things in the sport. Fate, however, had other ideas.

First Signs of Trouble

In 2014, I played my first year of senior footy for Crib Point Football Club. Due to my height and size, they put me in full back, which I adapted to quickly. I'd look at my opponents and think, *You can't beat me.* That was my mindset. No one was ever going to beat me, and, for the most part, no one did. We won game after game and eventually made the grand final. Duane Annable was our coach, and he was unreal. The passion he had for his players and the club was immense. He taught us to trust in our abilities, and, knowing he had our backs, we developed a level of confidence and passion that made us stand a little taller. I truly believe the success and drive of our team stemmed from his ability to make each player play at their best. We ended up losing that grand final game, but we didn't let it bring us down. Overall, we knew we'd had a great season and made our club proud.

It was a memorable time in my life. I felt so free. Perhaps that's mainly in comparison to my current lifestyle, but they really were good times. The club felt alive – it was thriving. I'd never experienced anything like it before. Everyone was so happy. We were all playing with mates, attending functions, and enjoying our success. Random people would approach us, shake our hands, say, "Good game," and shout us beers.

After every home game, we had to pick up rubbish that the spectators had left around the ground. But do you know what? It didn't bother us. We were pumped from winning and drinking the free beer our members bought us. Life was awesome and seemed like it would only get better.

I had two good years of seniors before the back issues started.

A Promising Career Cut Short

In my third year of seniors' football, I started getting mild back pain. At least, it was only mild at first. Eventually, it began to affect my performance on the field.

Initially, I tried to address the issue by getting a rub at three-quarter time, which helped a little. Four games later, I was getting a rub at half-time. Four games after that, I'd need a rub at quarter time, half-time, three-quarter time, and after the game. While I couldn't give 100 percent on the field, I was able to get through the games. However, the pain was getting worse, and, if I didn't work out what the hell was going on, it wouldn't be long before I could no longer make it through an entire game.

As the pain progressed, I saw a physio, a myotherapist, and a chiropractor, trying to understand and fix the problem. They all had answers – tight hamstrings, hard ground – but none of their explanations led to a solution. Soon, even with three separate professionals on the job, several months had passed, and the pain had only got worse. Finally, I went for an MRI at Frankston Hospital and discovered the source of the issue.

I'd never heard of autoimmune disease before. Growing up, I'd never been seriously sick, never had a serious injury, and now the doctors were telling me I had something called an autoimmune disease. Initially, I was more confused than concerned. *An autoimmune disease? What's that?* All I knew was that something called autoimmunity was causing inflammation in my back, which, in turn, was causing the pain. Apparently, it was a bit more serious than tight hamstrings. But how much more serious?

Although autoimmune conditions are quite common, they aren't common in my family or friendship groups, and it took me a while to understand the situation.

The doctor explained, "The official term for what you have is ankylosing spondylitis."

"Is that bad?" I asked.

"For many people, it's manageable."

Great – if it's manageable, I'll learn to manage it. Simple, right?

Unfortunately, I had a tough decision to make. While footy was a big part of my life, it was absolutely contributing to the pain and inflammation. Could I give up the game I loved? My body answered the question for me. After a major flare up, I decided to quit footy and focus on managing my condition. Soon, making sacrifices for my health would be a constant reality.

By age 21, I'd played 53 senior football games. In fact, I never missed a game. I never got injured. Now, my own body was working against me, and I was forced to retire, in my mind, way too early.

Sport Was Great, but I Had Another Calling

As I mentioned, Dad was a carpenter. He was also my best friend growing up. He ran his own business and worked a lot of weekends, which was fine because I'd just spend time with him onsite. Like most kids, I loved building stuff, and the love never went away.

Dad used to frame houses, and I could often be seen climbing through the trusses like a monkey, which sometimes made the other workers nervous. He also used to fill up cans with sand, sit them on top of a fence, and set me up with an air fixing gun so I could get in some target practice. Clearly, Dad was pretty relaxed with me onsite, and I loved being there with him. Frankly, he was my hero.

Just like I wanted to make him proud with footy, I also wanted to make him proud with carpentry. I wanted to be as good as him. Really, I wanted to be just like him. So, when I was old enough, I helped out onsite on weekends and eventually began an apprenticeship with Dad's old apprentice, Tom, who'd started his own business. Regardless of the career I chose, Dad wanted me to finish school, so I attended VCAL (Victoria Certificate of Applied Learning) classes two days a week, graduating at age 17 and going straight into an apprenticeship. Seriously, I had maybe a one-week break before jumping into carpentry full-time. I literally went straight to work, skipping schoolies and using tools I got as Christmas presents.

To me, as a young man, starting an apprenticeship was exciting. I wasn't just trying to make Dad proud; I loved carpentry, and, of course, I liked the idea of making money and starting a career. I was passionate about the work, taking every opportunity to learn and grow. Eventually, I was running Tom's crew, picking the boys up in the work car and setting them up with tasks for the day. I also worked most weekends, building decks and pergolas, to make some extra money for tools and improve my skills quicker. When the time came to be signed off, I was more than ready to receive my official qualification and go out on my own.

Treatment, Management, Hope for a Cure

While my autoimmune condition forced me to quit footy, I was still relatively okay at work. The job was quite physical, but it wasn't like I was running, jumping, and twisting like I was on the footy field, and I was able to stay on the tools. Sure, I was still in pain, but it was manageable. At work, I could control the way I moved a lot more, and, while I was stiff and sore at the end of most days, the pain wasn't debilitating. Besides, I'd already given up on one dream, and I wouldn't sacrifice another so easily.

The first step in treating my autoimmune disease was to reduce the physical stress on my body. *Done.* The next step was to find a healer.

My stepmum, Monique, recommended that I see a naturopath to try to fix my autoimmune disease. *What the hell's a naturopath?* I didn't know anything about natural or alternative medicine, but, at that point, I was willing to give anything a go. It's a mindset I'm glad I adopted early on. Without a willingness to be open-minded and explore alternative solutions, my journey could've taken a completely different turn. Besides, who wants to be in constant pain? I wanted to fix my autoimmune disease and get on with my life, whatever it took. If my condition got worse, it could spread to other parts of my body and cause joints to seize. Well, I didn't want that, so I gave naturopathy a shot, booking an appointment with Sheryl, who came highly recommended.

After learning more about my condition, she suggested several lifestyle changes, the main one being a change in diet. I needed to reduce inflammation in my body, so, at Sheryl's recommendation, I became vegetarian and adopted a low-inflammatory diet. Why? Because my stomach was struggling to digest meat, which meant my body was using unnecessary energy for digestion that could've been directed at healing the autoimmune problems. It may not be the right diet for everyone – we're all different – but it has worked for me. Essentially, the goal was to keep my body as clean as possible so it could focus on healing.

I also started taking natural anti-inflammatory supplements. I don't recall exactly what they were, but I know one included turmeric. On top of that, I did kinesiology, acupuncture, chiropractic, some emotional work – anything that might help.

Overall, the treatments and lifestyle changes did improve my condition, and I was successfully managing the pain while continuing to work in my carpentry business. I hadn't cured the condition; the pain still lingered, but I was living a relatively normal life. Eventually, I decided to jump back on the footy field for one game in the reserves.

What could possibly go wrong?

ZACK'S HEALTH AND WELLBEING TIP

SUPPORT YOUR BODY WITH SUPPLEMENTS

If you're suffering with any health issue, whether it be inflammation, poor sleep, low energy, depression, or something else, supplements may complement relevant lifestyle changes.

In my case, anti-inflammatory supplements, such as turmeric, helped support my body to manage my autoimmune condition. Curcumin, a compound found in turmeric, has been scientifically proven to reduce inflammation.[1] When choosing supplements, it's important to do so with the guidance of a professional, whether that be a medical doctor, naturopath, or other health practitioner. Alternatively, if you're comfortable, you can do your own research, ensuring you're aware of any potential side effects.

While supplements won't necessarily cure a condition, they can support our bodies to heal and function at their best.

#1

"

Character cannot be developed in ease and quiet. Only through experience of trial and suffering can the soul be strengthened, vision cleared, ambition inspired, and success achieved.

– HELEN KELLER

Chapter 2

THE REAL STRUGGLE BEGINS

Trigger Point

My one-game return to footy took place in the reserves team. It was on a Friday night, and I didn't plan to play too hard. My back was still a major issue, and I'd need rubs every quarter to keep going. The plan was to sit at full forward the entire game, which I did for the first quarter, but I couldn't help myself. I wanted to get my hands dirty, so I put myself in the guts and ended up playing a good game. After so much time off the field, it was nice to be running around again, and, aside from a sore knee, I felt okay. That, however, would soon change.

My knee, which stayed sore for days afterwards, eventually grew a slight lump. *That's weird.* To try to get the inflammation down, I decided I'd bathe in the ocean every night. So, every night, I went down to the beach with my partner Tessa and my dog Fawn and soaked in the salt water, hoping the inflammation would subside.

A few days later, a lump appeared on my other knee. *What's happening?* Clearly, my body was having a flare up. At the time, I didn't understand how bad it would get.

From Bad to Unbearable

No matter what I did, the swelling didn't go down – it only got worse. It wasn't just the swelling that got worse but also the pain. Although it started in my knees, it quickly spread down my legs and to my feet. Eventually, the pain turned to agony. It felt like 1000 bees were stinging my feet, and it wouldn't stop. *Why won't it stop?*

As far as I could tell, my immune system had gone into overdrive, attacking my legs as if they were the enemy. *Why's this happening?* I didn't know. Perhaps the run on the footy field had contributed. Or maybe it was just a random flare up. The uncertainty I felt at that point would become a constant feature of the journey ahead.

The pain was excruciating, some of the worst I'd ever felt – and that's saying something. I've got tattoos all over my body, so I'd been pushed to what I thought was my pain threshold many times over. The pain now was unbearable. I wasn't quite screaming out in agony, but I was close. No matter what I did, the pain wouldn't stop, and I was quickly approaching breaking point. Standing was torture, and sleeping was near-impossible. At night, Tessa would rub my feet to help me get to sleep, which did help a little, but the pain never faded. It was always there, tormenting me every second of the day.

For over a week, I tried to persevere, pushing through the discomfort, hoping my body would sort itself out, but it never did. The swelling in my legs just kept getting worse. I know I should have seen a doctor when it got really bad, but

I hate hospitals, and I wanted to avoid stepping foot in one unless it was absolutely necessary. Eventually, it did become necessary. The pain was so overwhelming, so constant, so relentless that I couldn't take it anymore. At that point, I would've done anything to make it stop. I couldn't handle another day of constant agony. I'd take any pill, undergo any procedure, do whatever it took to stop the pain.

It was Mum who gave me the final push I needed to seek help. "Get in the car," she said. "We're going to Frankston." At that point, I didn't have the strength to argue, so I agreed, and she drove me to Frankston Hospital.

After being admitted, I underwent a series of scans to try to figure out what was happening. Previously, the pain and inflammation had only been in my back, but now, as I well knew, it had spread to other parts of my body. Eventually, we had an answer as to *what* was happening, although it wasn't immediately clear *why*.

Basically, inflammation within my body had gone into overdrive, and my immune system was attacking my bones in my legs and feet, causing the swelling and pain. Inflammation in general isn't bad. It's a part of the body's healing response. For instance, if we cut ourselves or get an infection, the immune system responds with inflammation to help fix or fight off the problem. In my case, however, the immune system was targeting areas of the body that didn't need healing, flooding my joints with inflammation, resulting in constant, agonising pain. Because there was nothing to heal, the immune response didn't stop – it didn't know *when* to stop – so it just kept going, and going, and going. Basically, my immune system was stuck in attack mode with no way to know the battle was over. Finally, I had a diagnosis of sorts, or at least an explanation for the swelling and pain. The next step was treatment.

No Treatment Option Was Off the Table

As a first step, the nurses stuck needles in my knees and drained some of the fluid. It wasn't exactly a pleasant experience, but I'd do whatever it took to stop the agony. A few needle pricks were just a drop in the ocean of pain I was feeling.

They weren't able to drain the fluid from my feet or ankles, but they did shoot them full of cortisone to reduce the inflammation. The treatment worked, but only for a few days. Quickly, the pain and swelling returned, and I had to search for alternative solutions. That's when I learnt about faecal transplants.

If you've never heard of faecal transplants, let me explain. Basically, they take donor poo from a healthy person and transplant it into someone else. Once transplanted into the top of the colon, good bacteria from the healthy poo spreads throughout the gut to help strengthen the internal microbiome. In my case, we hoped it would help reduce the inflammation.

My naturopath, Sheryl, suggested I undergo a faecal transplant with Dr Froomes, a gastroenterologist, after we traced my autoimmune issue to a possible cause: an over-growth of a bacteria called Klebsiella in the gut. Klebsiella, as it turns out, has a direct link to ankylosing spondylitis. The overgrowth had likely taken place over several months, if not years, with symptoms presenting over time. Another possible trigger was stress. Of course, the autoimmune issue itself did cause some stress, which may well have contributed to the major flare up.

So, back to the faecal transplant.

In normal circumstances, I would've been hesitant to agree to have a piece of foreign poo inserted into my colon – I'd never even heard of a faecal transplant before – but I was desperate for a cure, so I went along with the procedure.

Before the transplant, I needed to kill off the Klebsiella and other bad bacteria in my gut. The solution was a full week of heavy antibiotics, ensuring that nothing, good or bad, was left alive. After that, I had to drink a salt-water-like solution to flush out my system. Next, they transplanted the donor poo into my colon. Because the poo was frozen, it wasn't as effective as a fresh sample would've been. As they say, fresh is always better than frozen. What did this mean? Well, for me, it meant that I had to drive to the hospital every day to have fresh poo inserted into my colon. Thankfully, Mum, my guardian angel, offered to drive me each day, as the trip was an hour and a half each way and I was still recovering from my flare up. Our goal was to get my gut healthy again and halt the out-of-control autoimmune response, and I was grateful for the support, something I'd soon need a lot more of.

On top of the faecal transplant, I also had to receive daily enemas, which, again, Mum helped with. In the end, she practically became my full-time nurse. The faecal transplants were very vulnerable moments, having to stick a pipe up there to implant good bacteria in my gut. But I knew that if I stayed strong and completed the ten-day transplant and enema protocol, I had a good chance of recovery. With that in mind, I persevered and made it through to the end of the treatment.

Hope on the Horizon

Within two weeks, the inflammation had gone down by about 50 percent, and I was able to get around on crutches.

Eventually, I was able to ditch the crutches altogether and walk unassisted. The faecal transplant had worked its magic, and it seemed that I was on track to recovery.

During this time, I lost a lot of weight. Have you ever been in so much pain you can't eat? That's how I felt during the worst of the flare up – too sick to eat. Before the flare up, I weighed around 95 kg. By the time the symptoms began to ease, I'd dropped down to about 75 kg. That's a 20 kg drop in weight in only a month. I also looked very pale – you could tell I was unwell just by looking at me. Being in pain 24/7 drains the life out of you, making it difficult to function.

During my recovery, I really pushed the alternative therapies, using anything I could get my hands on to help my body heal. For me, it was a process of rebuilding after the autoimmune flare up had broken me down.

As well as following Sheryl's advice, I booked a wellness retreat on the Gold Coast and brought my partner in crime Tessa with me. I sought the expertise of a health guru named Don Tolman, who recommended water fasting, among other diets and natural remedies. For me, fasting was a game changer. With that said, the first three days – out of a ten-day fast – were rough. I experienced body soreness and some pretty severe headaches. At one point, it felt like I had termites in my head. My body wanted me to quit, but I pushed through, and soon the positive effects began to show. When you're taking on any big challenge, whether it be fasting, running a marathon, or undergoing difficult medical treatment, it's important to remember why you're doing it. The first three days without food nearly broke me, but I made it through to earn the benefits. When you're ready to quit, keep the outcome in mind. Keep hold of your why. There's a good chance you're stronger than you think.

Surprisingly, when I wasn't taking in any food, I didn't feel any pain. It was as if my body was using the inflammation as energy, burning it away and relieving the pressure. I returned to work and was able to go all day relatively pain-free. It helped that I was keeping my mind busy so I wasn't focusing on the pain. Because I was fasting, my body didn't need to use resources digesting food, so it was able to focus on healing the inflammation, and it worked wonders. Surprisingly, my energy levels were still pretty good, even though I was consuming nothing but water. It's amazing how the body can adapt to changing circumstances.

On day ten of the water fast, I started introducing cold-pressed juices into my diet. I wasn't just blending fruit; I bought an actual cold-press juicer and made the juices fresh each day. Because my body had been so long without food, I couldn't just end the fast with a big feed of Maccas or anything like that. Instead, I had to slowly reintroduce foods, starting with juices and broths. I'd make up four or five juices in the mornings and sip on them throughout the day, gradually bringing my digestive system back online. I was working on the tools full-time, which kept my mind off food for the majority of the day.

The energy the juice gave me was unreal. After ten days of no food, the natural sugars in the fruit practically got me high. I felt so clean and pure. Because I hadn't reintroduced heavier foods yet, my body processed the juice quickly and cleanly, absorbing all the good stuff, all the nutrients.

The next phase involved introducing soups into my diet, continuing to ease my stomach back into digesting heavier foods. Soon, I fully returned to my vegetarian diet, with my body feeling much better than it had when I first started fasting. However, I wasn't completely recovered. Some of the inflammation remained, and none of the alternative treatments I was trying seemed capable of clearing it out. I was so close to fully recovered, but I couldn't quite get across the line. *What now?*

Out of desperation, I turned back to conventional medicine and made what may well have been the biggest mistake of my life.

ZACK'S HEALTH AND WELLBEING TIP

USE FASTING TO HEAL AND REBOOT YOUR BODY

Water fasting, the type I used to combat my auto-immunity, has several reported health benefits, including improved general health and lowered risk of chronic disease.[2] Sounds great, right?

For me, it worked wonders, but you don't need to take the extreme approach I did to reap the benefits of fasting. Even intermittent fasting, where you consistently fast for a set chunk of the day – for example, a 16-hour window – can positively affect your health.[3]

Of course, you should always consult a professional before adding fasting to your routine.

#2

"

It is your reaction
to adversity, not
the adversity itself,
that determines
how your life's
story will develop.

– DIETER F. UCHTDORF

Chapter 3

RED FLAGS
AS FAR AS
THE EYE
CAN SEE

Willing to Try Anything

When the doctors at the hospital offered me HUMIRA, I didn't know much about the medication. As it was explained to me, the drug works by suppressing the immune system, slowing it down when it's overactive and attacking things it shouldn't. At this point, I was keen to try anything that would help me get better. Besides, it was just some lingering inflammation I wanted to get rid of. No big deal, right? While I was still in some pain after the faecal transplant, the treatment had done its job, and my latest blood test showed that my inflammatory markers had notably reduced. In fact, they'd reduced to a point where I wasn't actually eligible for a HUMIRA injection. But I was still in pain. Most days, it felt like termites were eating away at my joints, which, to be fair, was an improvement on the 1000 bee stings, but still not ideal.

When they said I wasn't eligible for the medication, I thought I was out of options, until the doctor explained that we could use the results of a previous blood test, which showed higher levels of inflammation. Based on those results, we could go ahead with the HUMIRA injection. Looking back, the whole interaction was a massive red flag.

I was, of course, aware of the risks. Most, if not all, medications come with side effects. Even if you pick up a common drug, like Panadol for instance, and read the box, you're going to see a list of nasty side effects. So, when I was told that HUMIRA can increase the risk of developing certain cancers, I assumed the risk was low and I'd be okay.[4] *Plenty of people take the medication, and they're fine. Why would I be any different?*

Risk vs. Reward

It's easy to look back and say, "I should have done this," or, "I shouldn't have done that," but, at the time, I was simply doing what I thought was best for me, my body, and my recovery. I knew a guy who'd been on the drug for years and was still able to play local footy. *What if I respond well to the treatment? What if I can play footy again? What if I can get my life back?* At the time, the potential rewards outweighed the stated risks. I've since changed that opinion.

Because I was being prescribed the medication outside of normal circumstances, the treatment protocol was a bit experimental, and the doctors monitored me closely, frequently checking my response and inflammation levels.

HUMIRA is delivered via a tiny needle, like an insulin injection, into the stomach. It's a simple delivery, but I felt anxious every time, the possible risks always on my mind. I decided I wouldn't accept being on the drug long-term; I just wanted to get my body back to a healthy baseline.

Over the next couple of months, I continued to take the HUMIRA as prescribed and saw my symptoms improve. Eventually, I got to a point where I no longer needed the injections, and I stopped taking HUMIRA altogether. At that point, I was feeling pretty good and was relieved to be done with the treatment. Finally, things were looking up. Being me, I had done everything in my power to heal, which meant combining the faecal transplants with the injections. The strategy had paid off – my inflammatory markers were low. Unfortunately, they might have been too low.

Taking Care of Business

Now that I was successfully managing my autoimmune issue, I was free to focus on one of my great loves: carpentry. I jumped into action, putting on two new apprentices and getting back to work. I'd worked hard to get where I was, and my business was doing well. I could accept losing footy, but I'd hold on to carpentry with all my might.

When my autoimmune disease first surfaced and I was experiencing back pain, I worked through the discomfort. It helped that I loved carpentry, but I also had a house to pay off, so I pushed through the pain. When the big flare up struck, I was off my feet for a few months, and working wasn't an option. I was tough; I was resilient, but I had my limits. I needed to take time to heal. When you're dealing with adversity, it's important to know which battles to fight. Could I have pushed through the pain and continued to work? Maybe, but I don't imagine my workmanship would've been topnotch. Sometimes taking a step back is the smart move.

Once I got on top of the pain, I was straight back on the tools, doing what I loved. I was still building myself back up, regaining the weight I'd lost, but I was in relatively good shape. Or so I thought.

It's Just a Lump...

About eight months after returning to work, something strange happened. I found a lump on my shin. I didn't think much of it at first. I assumed it was connected to the auto-immune stuff and would eventually go down. Or maybe it was a cyst that I'd need to get cut out. It wasn't painful; I wasn't peeing blood, and I wasn't experiencing any other symptoms, just the lump itself.

For a while, I completely ignored it. I was, after all, busy running a business. I was also going to the gym, trying to build my body back up again, and I didn't notice any decline in health. As far as I knew, everything was fine.

Over time, I noticed that the lump wasn't shrinking. *Hm… that's strange.* But I was too flat out at work to give it much thought. See, I'm not a worry wart. In my mind, I'd eventually get the lump checked; it would turn out to be a cyst; they'd buzz it off, and I'd get on with my life, no dramas. Thankfully, Tessa was the voice of reason, and she kept urging me to get it checked. Finally, I agreed.

A Quick Fix, I Thought

One night after work, I went for an ultrasound at a nearby imaging centre. I thought I knew exactly how it would play out. First, they'd do the scan and tell me I had a cyst. Next, they'd book me in for surgery, and I'd have it shaved off. Simple, right? I was way off.

During the ultrasound, I noticed that the technician was staring at the screen with a look of concern. Something told me he didn't think it was a cyst.

"What is it?" I asked.

"I'm just trying to rule out a blood clot," he said.

Blood clot? I knew that a blood clot, if serious enough, could lead to losing a limb. *Are they about to tell me I'm going to lose my leg?*

"Is it serious?" I asked.

"Oh, no, not usually. We can treat most blood clots with blood thinners."

That's a relief.

"We're going to need to do another scan to confirm exactly what it is."

"Okay," I said. "When can I book it in?"

"We'll do it right now," the technician said.

That's when it hit me that something was wrong. A big red flag. How often does someone get a scan so quickly – immediately? Unfortunately, our healthcare system isn't that efficient. Suddenly, however, I was at the front of the queue, being rushed into the next room for an emergency contrast CT scan.

I received a dye injection – the type that makes you feel like you're about to pee your pants – let it sit in my body for 15 minutes, and then had the scan. Once the scan was over, I walked through to where the technicians were looking at their screens.

"So, what is it?" I asked. "Is it a blood clot?"

"Um, we can't give you the full report right now… but unfortunately it looks like a tumour."

I paused as I processed what he'd said. "What?"

"Oh, but tumours can be benign. We've just got to rule out that it's cancerous."

Shit… It has to be benign, right?

"The doctor will call you with the results tonight."

With nothing left to do but wait, I walked outside, and the possibility of cancer really started to hit home. It was about 6 pm, and I didn't know what to do, so I called Mum, and then Dad, explaining the situation.

"I've got a tumour," I told Dad, "but they don't know if it's cancerous or benign… I could have cancer." At that point, I was getting pretty worked up. Either I had cancer, or I had nothing – two very different possibilities.

"Calm down, mate, you can get benign tumours. You'll be all right." He was right. I had no reason to believe that the tumour was cancerous, so there was no reason to get worked up about it. After all, cancer didn't run in the family, and I felt fairly healthy – it wasn't like I was coughing up blood – so a benign tumour seemed the most likely diagnosis.

With a more positive mindset, I drove home to wait for the doctor's call.

Incoming Call...

Thankfully, I didn't have to wait alone. Tessa was there with me, and Mum and my stepdad Deane came over to support me as well.

We were all sitting in the lounge room, talking, when the call came in. Suddenly, everyone was silent. I went over to the kitchen bench to take the call.

"Hello."

"Zack Condick?"

"Yeah."

"The results of the contrast CT scan show you've got a bone sarcoma, a malignant tumour. You should go straight to emergency and start treatment right away."

What? Since when do you go to emergency for cancer? I couldn't make sense of what was happening. *Emergency? Fuck, is he saying it's spreading by the second?* I didn't have a doctor who I saw regularly – until the autoimmune issue, I'd rarely been sick – so the guy on the other end of the phone was just whichever bulk-billing doctor happened to be available at the time. He didn't know me, and it seemed that his only goal was to deliver the bad news and get off the phone as quickly as possible.

I ended the call, dropping the phone. "I'm fucked." Everyone was watching me, waiting for an explanation. "He said I've got a cancerous tumour." Everyone in the room broke down, and, for me, the panic started to kick in.

My life had just changed in a way I was yet to fully comprehend.

ZACK'S HEALTH AND WELLBEING TIP

FINE-TUNE YOUR DIET

When my autoimmune disease first flared up, I switched to a vegetarian diet to help lower inflammation. The switch was very purposeful, as my body wasn't digesting meat well.

If you're experiencing any health issues, it's worth seeing what you can adjust in your diet to help alleviate symptoms. I'm not saying everyone should be vegetarian, but making dietary changes, especially if certain foods are causing a negative reaction, can have a profound impact on our overall health. For example, if a gluten allergy is causing inflammation in the gut, removing gluten from your diet would be beneficial.

At the very least, we should aim to eat as cleanly as possible as often as possible, because a healthy diet is a critical component of good health.[5]

#3

"

I've got a theory
that if you give
100 percent all of
the time, somehow
things will work
out in the end.

– LARRY BIRD

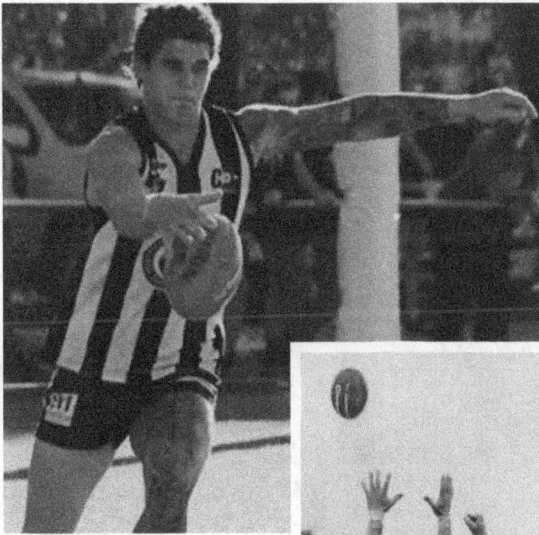

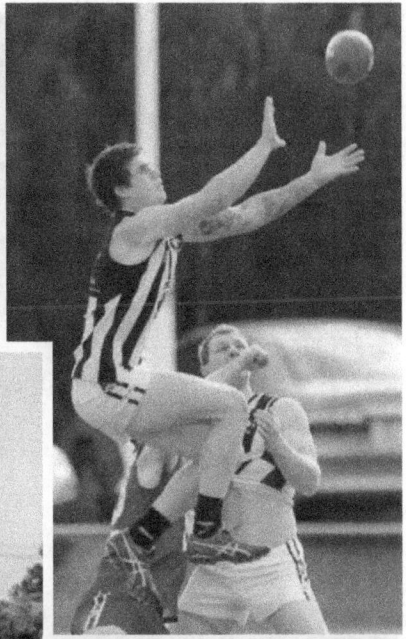

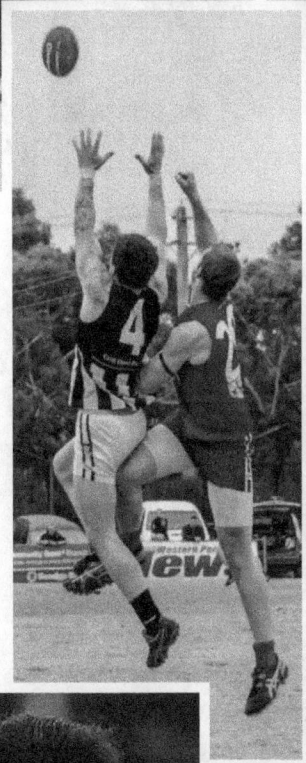

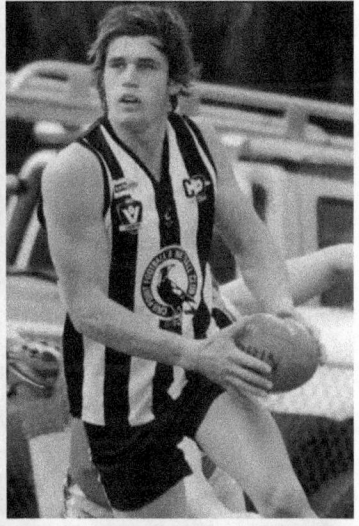

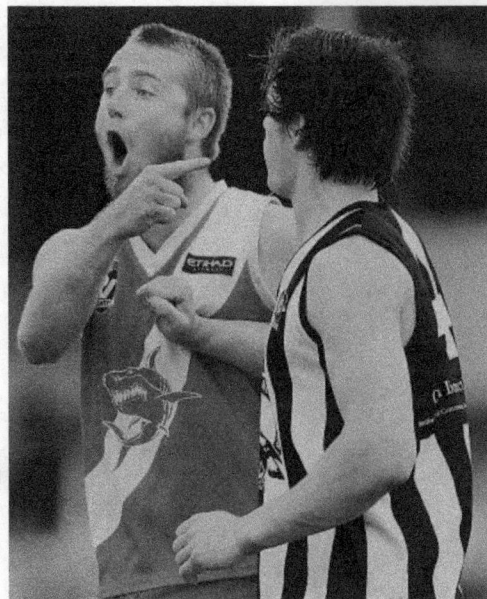

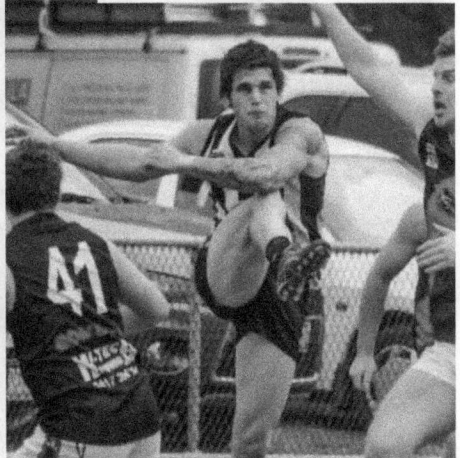

Zack playing
seniors footy
for Crib Point
Football Club
2014–2015.

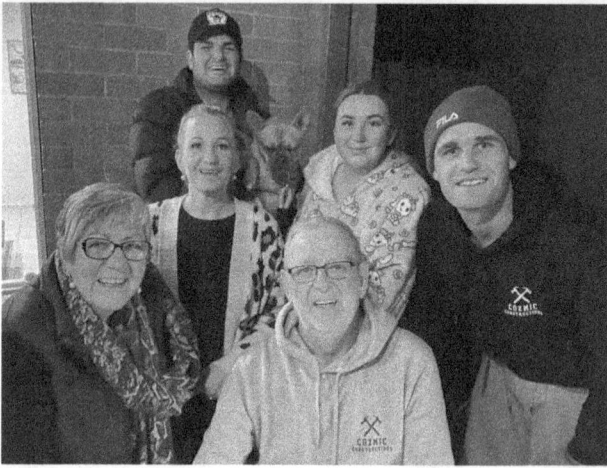

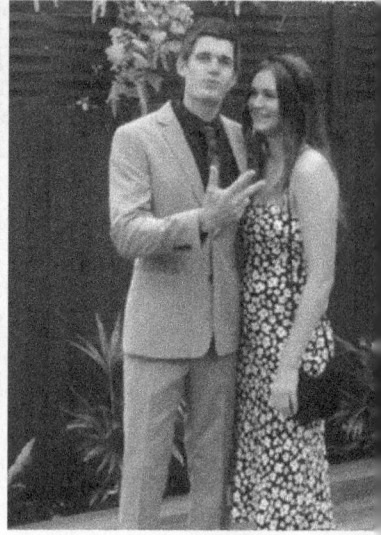

Good times with loved ones.

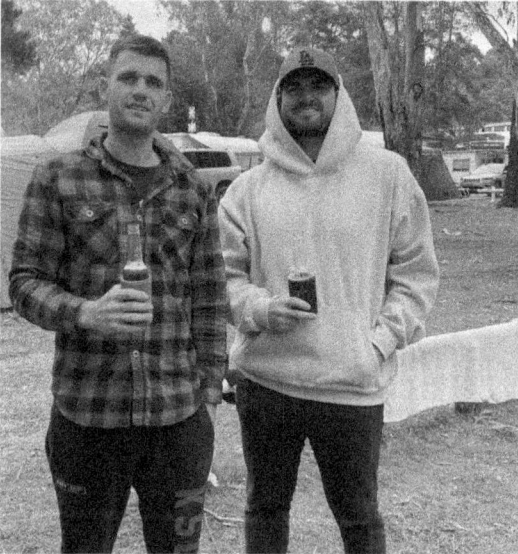

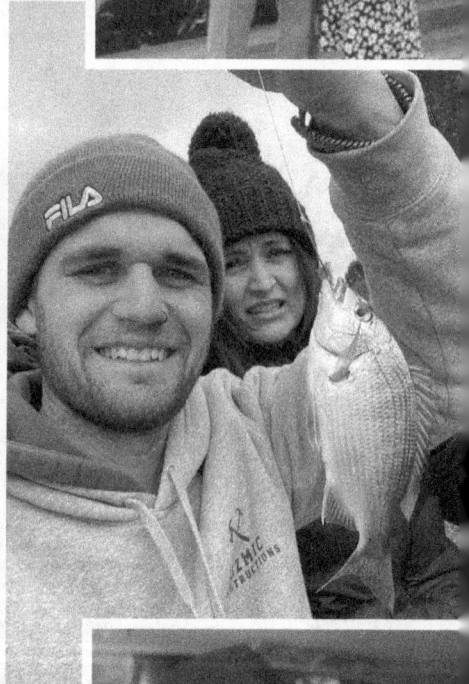

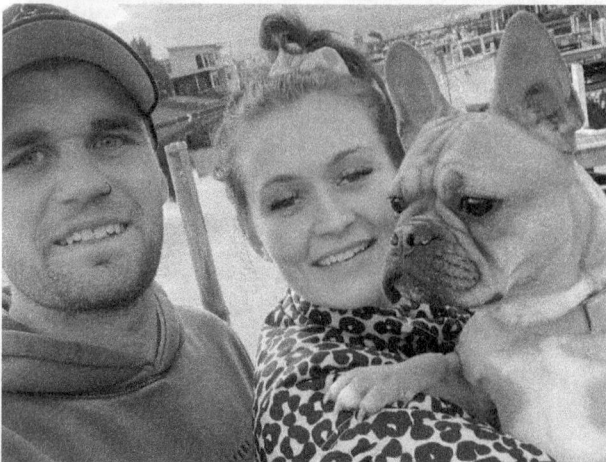

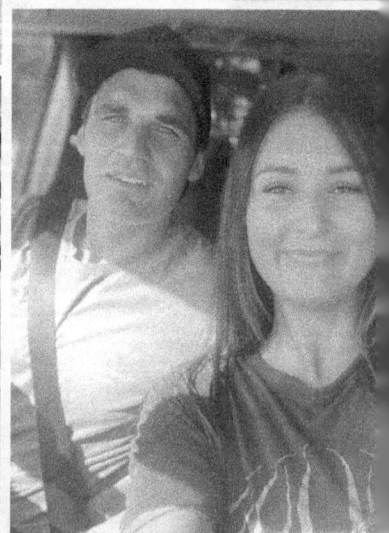

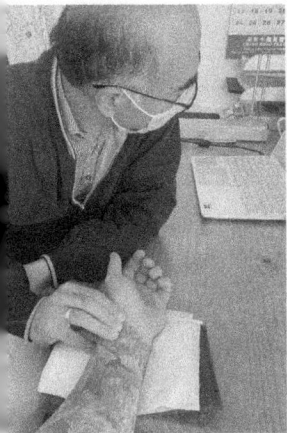

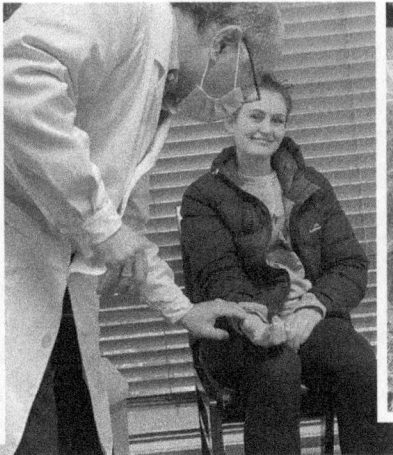

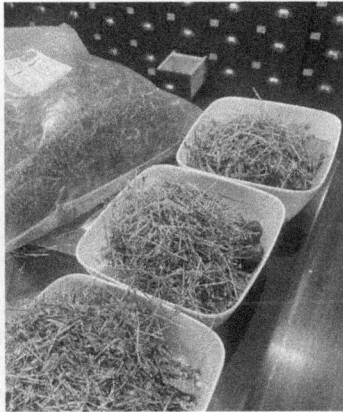

Master and his Chinese medicinal herbs.

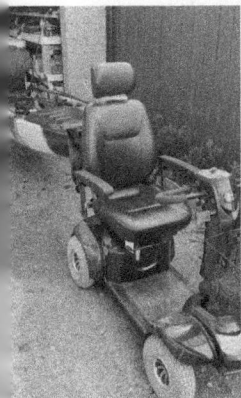

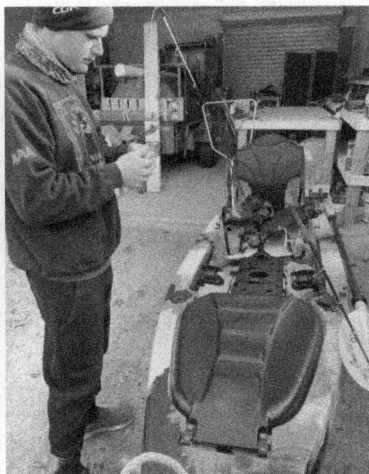

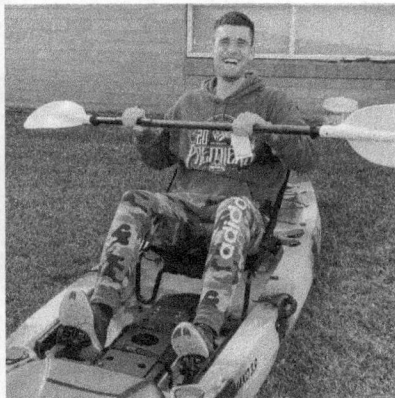

New fishing kayak gifted by good mates.

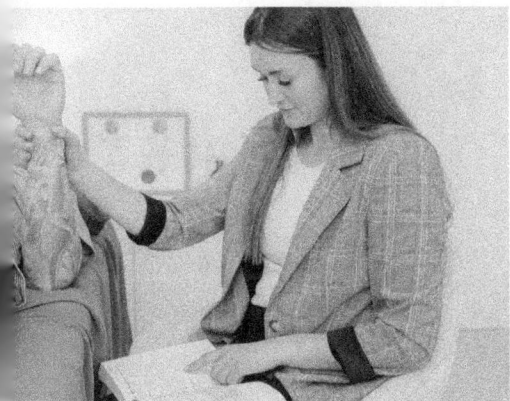

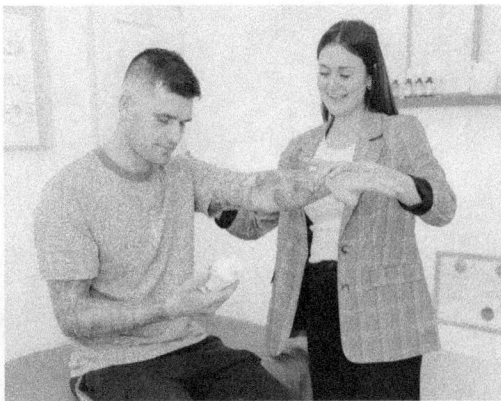

Tessa giving Zack a check-up at her wellness centre, Align Wellness Studio.

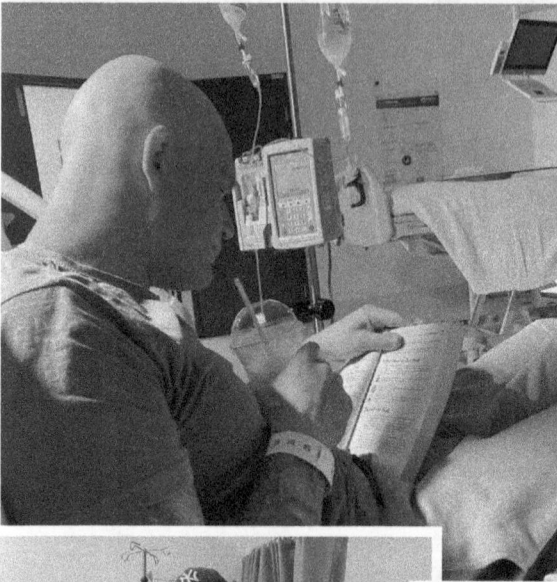

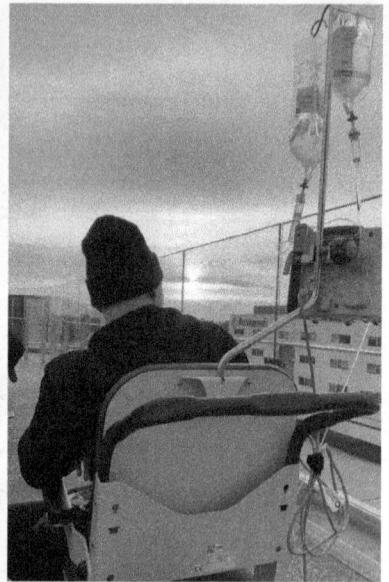

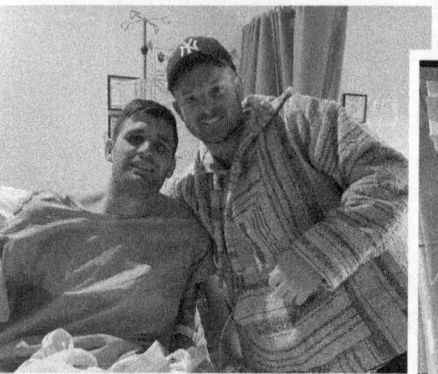

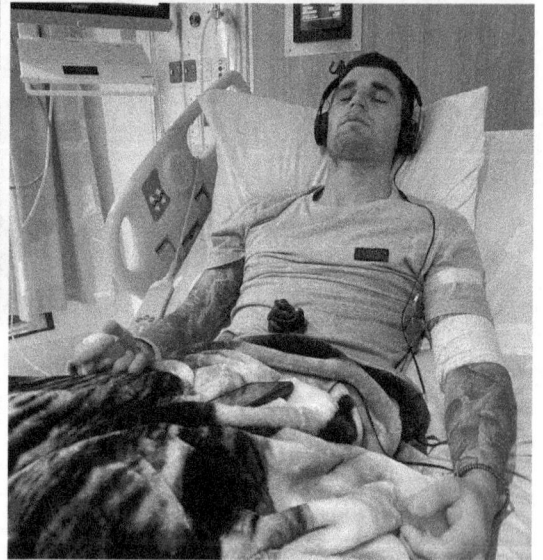

Zack undergoing treatment
at Peter Mac and St Vincent's
hospitals.

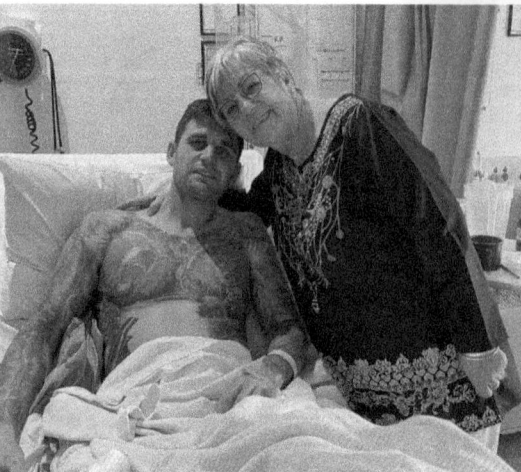

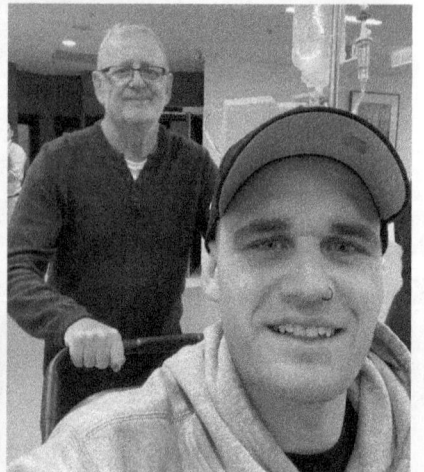

Chapter 4

DETERMINED TO FIGHT

And So It Begins

After my cancer diagnosis, I saw another doctor, who referred me to the Peter MacCallum Cancer Centre, also known as 'Peter Mac', the best cancer hospital in our state and possibly our whole country. Yet it was troubling to learn that only serious, life-threatening cases go there. Despite what the doctor on the phone had suggested, I didn't end up going to emergency. I'm not entirely sure why he told me to do that.

As a first step in the treatment process, I was scheduled to undergo a series of scans and procedures at Peter Mac. I'd never known anyone with cancer, so I had no idea what I was in for or what I was up against.

Surrendering to the System

Before I could begin treatment, or even know if treatment was possible, the doctors had to determine what type of cancer I had. Different cancers require different treatments, and apparently there are 160 different types of bone sarcomas. Some require radiation, while others require chemo. Some require a combination of both.

To find out what type of cancer I had, I needed to have a biopsy, which would involve puncturing the tumour and taking a sample. I'll admit, the procedure made me nervous. *What if puncturing the tumour releases the cancer into other parts of my body? Isn't that a thing? Isn't that what kills some people?* Like I said, I had no experience with cancer, so I was constantly trying to determine whether the doctors were taking the right approach or not. While I'll never know if the HUMIRA caused the cancer, I couldn't help but wonder, and I didn't want to make another potentially fatal mistake. I wanted to trust the experts, but, naturally, I was hesitant.

When I voiced my concerns about puncturing the tumour, the doctors admitted there was some risk of spreading the cancer if the biopsy went wrong. They also said they wouldn't know how to treat it without learning what they were dealing with.

At that point, I realised, if I wanted to beat the cancer, I had no choice but to surrender myself to the medical system and trust in the expertise of the doctors. Among all the uncertainty, I just had to have faith.

Preparing for War

When I found out I had cancer, I went and saw Sheryl right away, and she sprang into action, putting me on a diet that consisted of nothing but boiled greens – bok choy, broccoli, things like that. The theory was that the greens would be easy on my digestive system so my body could concentrate on attacking the cancerous tumour, while still providing the nutrients my body needed to fight the cancer. For several months, that's all I ate. Boiled greens. Every. Single. Day. I also drank food-grade hydrogen peroxide 35 percent daily, which was like pouring turps down my throat, but I was determined to do whatever it took to kill the lump.

I also did a two-week water fast. I knew from my experience with the autoimmune issue that fasting would give my body the break it needed to focus on attacking the tumour.

But I didn't stop there. I fully intended to throw everything available at the lump on my leg. I never referred to it as 'cancer' – I didn't want to give it that sort of power. In my mind, it was just a lump, and it would soon be gone.

To complement everything else, Sheryl referred me to a Chinese doctor named Master. As he explained his process, including the herbs I'd be taking, he was very calm and collected. He'd dealt with plenty of life-threatening conditions before and didn't seem too worried, which was a relief. Even if his confidence was misguided, it helped boost my own. I needed every positive charge I could get.

Part of Master's treatment protocol involved Qigong healings, where he placed his hands on the tumour and used his chi energy to try to shrink it. Hey, I was willing to try anything at this point. If there was even the slightest chance that something would help, I was all for it.

Soon, I'd either be starting chemo or radiation, which I understood could be brutal on the body. However, with a solid alternative treatment plan in place, I was much better equipped for what lay ahead. Master and Sheryl had done everything in their power to prepare my body for the fight of my life.

Making It Official

Once the doctors had identified the type of cancer I had, I underwent a scan to find out exactly where the cancerous cells were and to see how active my tumour was. For the scan, I was injected with a radioactive substance, which came in what looked like a mini hand grenade with smoke coming off it. From the grenade, they pulled out the needle containing the radioactive contrast to inject into my body, making the cancer cells visible on the scanner. Apparently, it was only a small amount of radiation and wasn't cause for concern. Once again, I had to trust in the process. After they injected the radiation, I had to wait for an hour, sitting dead still, with no phone, no TV, until the substance had spread through my entire body. Apparently, electronics could stimulate certain parts of the body and cause inaccuracies on the scan. So, I sat in a reclining chair on one of the upper floors of Peter Mac, looking out over the city of Melbourne, wondering if my time was up. I reflected on my achievements and thought of my beautiful family. I had led a good life, but I wasn't ready for it to end just yet, so I prayed to God, asking for another chance and help with the fight ahead.

I wasn't the only cancer patient in that upper-floor room, either. Looking to the side, I saw at least six other people undergoing the same procedure, sitting, waiting, hoping. We were all there for the same reason. We all had a battle to fight. We all had cancer. It felt like a warzone, all of us sick, injured, fighting to survive. However, the real battle was just beginning.

Through the scan, doctors were able to identify the exact location and size of the tumour and see whether the cancer had spread to other parts of my body. The problem was, I didn't get the results until several days later, and I was left wondering, worrying, uncertain about how big of a fight I had on my hands. At that point, I didn't even know if I'd be undergoing treatment or if I only had three months to live. I was stuck in limbo.

On the same day, I had to have a PICC (peripherally inserted central catheter) line inserted, which is a pretty daunting procedure. If you're not aware, a PICC line is a thin tube that enters a vein in the arm and goes all the way to the heart. Why did I need such a thing? Well, the chemo-therapy medication was too strong to go directly into my veins – they would basically disintegrate before I could even finish my treatment – so it had to be directed right to my heart valve. Full on, I know.

Right before the procedure, which I'd be completely awake for, I was taken to a waiting room. Tessa sat next to me, holding my hand, but she wouldn't be allowed to enter the theatre. When my name was called, I put on my brave face and told her I'd be okay. Once we'd said what we needed to say to each other, I walked through the glass doors to the operating theatre, then stopped, turned back, saw Tessa watching me through the glass, and blew her a kiss. Then I was gone.

In the theatre, there were three doctors, screens every-where, and an operating table where I was told to lie down and make myself comfortable. Guided by ultrasound, the doctors inserted a metal wire into a vein in my arm and pushed it in as far as it would go, all the way to my heart. From memory, it went in roughly 50 cm. Next, they used the wire as a guide, pushing the catheter tube to my heart. Finally, they pulled the wire out and, with what was essen-tially a piece of sticky tape, covered the two valves protruding from my arm – one for delivering the chemo and another for flushing it out.

Now installed, the PICC line would stay inside me for the duration of my treatment. To me, it was symbolic. The PICC line officially marked me as a cancer patient.

The Real Fun Begins

Now that all the tests, scans, and procedures had been completed, it was time to start treatment – if treatment were possible. Before beginning chemo, I attended a meeting with several doctors at Peter Mac to discuss the next steps. Mum, Dad, and Tessa all came with me.

Firstly, the doctors explained that I had an osteosarcoma, a rare cancer that not many people survive. *Great.* Basically, I was given a 20 percent chance of living after chemo and surgery. After throwing everything modern medicine had at the lump, that was my chance of survival. A mere 20 percent. One in five. That's it. It's like rolling a five-sided dice and hoping to get a one. The odds weren't in my favour.

Surely, I must be due for some good news. It was wishful thinking. In reality, every time I thought the situation couldn't get any worse, it did, over and over again.

After giving my cancer a label, the doctors discussed the treatment plan – and it wasn't going to be pretty. They wanted to hit me with two of the strongest chemotherapy drugs around: methotrexate and doxorubicin. Over six months of treatment, in three-week cycles, I'd receive chemo for two days straight each cycle, followed by three days of flushing and two weeks at home to recover. If the chemicals weren't properly flushed from my system, my kidneys would fail. On top of that, for the five days per week I'd be receiving treatment, I'd need to stay in hospital so they could monitor me closely, as there was a risk of heart failure.

Then there was the surgery. Once the chemo had stopped the tumour from spreading and killed the cells inside it, the surgeons would need to cut whatever was left out of my leg, with big margins. Essentially, I'd be losing 22 cm of shinbone. Yep, more bad news. I'd never had a surgery before in my life, so the plan came as a bit of a shock. I assumed they'd replace the missing chunk of bone with a piece of metal, but that wasn't the case. Metal wasn't an option, as it wasn't strong enough and wouldn't last long, which, being so young, was a problem. If I was to walk again, I'd need to replace my missing shinbone with a new donor bone. *Okay, makes sense.* Oh, and the dead donor bone would need a live bone alongside it, so they'd need to remove the fibula from the same leg and use that. *The good news... it isn't coming, is it?*

Because there were so many opportunities for something to go wrong, I had to fill out forms detailing who could make decisions for me if I was no longer able. Just what I needed to shatter my confidence even further.

Oh, did I mention that the chemotherapy could very well make me infertile? Tessa and I did want to have kids one day, so I considered freezing my sperm. I was hit with so much information at once. It was a lot to take in. I was about to learn exactly what I was made of.

I took a deep breath. "Okay," I said, "when do we start chemo?"

"We should have started yesterday."

The Right Mindset for Survival

Although my treatment was urgent, there was a two-week gap before I started chemotherapy. Tessa and I thought about it long and hard, deciding that we wanted to have a kid no matter what. I had only a 20 percent chance of surviving, but I didn't want to believe that. I couldn't give in to that mindset; otherwise, the worst possible outcome would be more likely to become reality. Instead, I chose to live as if I was certain I'd survive.

We didn't expect anything to come of it, but Tessa and I tried for a baby during the two-week gap before chemo started. When undergoing chemotherapy, your body becomes super toxic. You're not even allowed to use the same toilet as other people, let alone have sexual intercourse. For the duration of my treatment, I'd practically be poison.

Reluctantly, I also went ahead and froze some sperm. Obviously, I was going through some heavy shit, and the last thing I wanted to do was go into the city and put sperm in a cup, but, in the end, I did what I had to do. Trust the process.

Focused on Healing

Before I started chemo, I saw some holistic healers and learnt about meditation and visualisation to help get me through the treatment. Remember, I was fully prepared to try everything possible to come out the other end alive. We're talking life or death here. Why wouldn't I want to give myself the best chance of survival?

Being injected with chemotherapy drugs is a distressing experience, so I wanted to do everything I could to keep my mind and body calm to better facilitate the healing process. As we know, stress itself can be a killer.

Deep down, I didn't want to do the chemo, and I felt resentful about the treatment, about feeling like I had no other choice. However, that mindset wouldn't help the healing process, so I had to shift to a more positive outlook. Visualisation was a part of the solution. Whenever I received chemo, as the drug travelled to my heart via the PICC line to be pumped throughout my body, I'd visualise it not as a poison but as a glowing, golden, healing liquid. It was there to help me, not harm me. I learnt not to fight it but instead to accept it and let it work its magic.

During treatment, I also wore earphones, often playing different meditations that Penny, my healer, had created for me. Sometimes I'd play calming rainforest sounds – anything to keep me calm and to block out the ceaseless, mind-numbing sound of the IV pump.

I even went as far as holding different healing crystals and a lucky Buddha, clutching to anything that might improve my odds of survival. All of this helped put me in a more positive mindset, the mindset I needed for healing.

From a physical perspective, I cut sugar out of my diet from day one, as sugar could feed the cancer, causing it to grow. In my mind, I was as prepared as I could possibly be. I'd seen chemotherapy in movies, and I knew it could be rough. Yes, I know movies aren't reality, but they were the only points of reference I had. The doctors also helped me understand what to expect as much as they could. Even so, I didn't fully understand how brutal chemotherapy could be until I'd lived it.

ZACK'S HEALTH AND WELLBEING TIP

PRACTISE VISUALISATION

Visualisation is a powerful tool anyone can use to help them achieve their goals. Leaders use it to get ahead; sports people use it to win, and many others use it in their daily lives.

In my case, visualisation helped me deal with a challenging situation. I also hoped it would help with the healing. The mind and body are closely connected, so I wanted to ensure my mind was working with me and not against me. At the very least, visualisation helped ease some of my anxiety.

If there's something you want to achieve, visualise it as if it's happening right now and get your brain and body on board. Visualisation isn't magic; you do still have to work for your goals, but it can boost your chances of succeeding.[6]

#4

"

If you're going through hell, keep going.

– WINSTON CHURCHILL

Chapter 5

WHEN THE CURE FEELS WORSE THAN THE DISEASE

Into the Fire

The first chemo session was a traumatic experience – I was shitting myself. They started with a small but strong dose of doxorubicin. While the IV bag was smaller than I'd expected, which should have been a relief, the colour of the chemical was off-putting – it was fluoro-red.

As the bright-red liquid made its way down the tube towards my arm, I closed my eyes and began my visualisation, imagining it with a golden glow. I was being healed, not hurt, and I focused on trying to believe that.

Every time I did the doxorubicin, there were four or five nurses in the room in case I had a heart attack, which was a real possibility with chemo that strong. The constant monitoring made getting into a meditative state very difficult. The first time was particularly difficult because no one knew how my body would react to the treatment. Heart attack, liver failure, death – they were all possibilities. Honestly, I didn't read too much into the worst possible side effects, as I didn't want them at the forefront of my mind. I didn't want to be sitting there, feel a pain in my chest, and automatically assume I was having a heart attack. I'm sure Mum and Tessa did more in-depth research, but I just needed to know enough to consent to the treatment.

At no point did I submit to having 'cancer'. It was always just a 'lump', a lump I needed to get rid of for myself and my family. My focus wasn't on what I had but instead on what I had to do to fix it – the alternative therapies, the chemo, the lifestyle changes.

I also stopped dwelling on the low chance of survival and how many people my type of lump had killed in the past. The survival rate didn't matter. All that mattered was surviving. I saw my family breaking down from my cancer journey, so I wasn't going to let it beat me. Not a chance. Instead, I stared death straight in the face and said, "Bring it on."

A Form of Torture

Once the doxorubicin entered my body, I started sweating, felt nauseous, and my face puffed up. Basically, I felt like absolute crap.

It only took 15 minutes to administer the entire dose. Once done, they switched me to a steroid drip with fluids to help flush out my system. Without it, the strong chemotherapy drug could've killed me.

So, for the rest of the day, I sat there, being pumped full of fluids, with the constant sound of the infusion pump drowning out everything around me. The machine, with its wheels and vertical pole that held the IV bags, never left me. Even if I had to go to the toilet or have a shower, I couldn't just put the pump on pause. I'd need to drag it along with me. If I wanted to go to the centre's rooftop café, the machine would need to come with me. If I needed to go *anywhere,* the machine came too. It was like a ball and chain. If I was trying to have a conversation with someone, I couldn't just turn down the pump's volume. It didn't work like that. Instead, we had to speak loudly to be heard. After a while, the continuous sound of the pump was like a subtle form of torture. I would put in my earphones and try to drown it out with music, but that only did so much. The sound was always there, reminding me where I was and what was happening.

On the second day, they pumped me full of the other chemo drug, methotrexate, which was clear in colour and took about one hour to administer. Then I spent the next three days having the chemotherapy drugs flushed from my system so my organs didn't fail from the treatment. It's a brutal way to treat a disease, but it was all the conventional medical system had to work with.

While sitting in my hospital room alone, I had a lot of thinking time. I'd often stare out my window, looking at the beautiful weather outside, thinking, *Please give me the strength to make it to the end.* I still had a long journey ahead of me.

When I was home for the two recovery weeks of my chemotherapy cycles, I couldn't enjoy my time away from the hospital, because I felt like absolute crap, like I'd been poisoned, which technically I had. I was like a zombie, shuffling to the pantry, forgetting why I was even there. Shuffling to another room, once again forgetting why. Chemo brain fog is real. At the time, I didn't know if the effects would be temporary or not. *Am I going to be brain damaged for the rest of my life?* Even though I tried to keep a positive attitude, those types of thoughts sometimes entered my mind, and I did my best to work through them.

Most days at home were a blur. I know I spent a lot of time on the couch, wrapped in a blanket, watching Netflix, but I don't remember what I watched. I don't think I was even paying attention. Most days, I just slept, or tried to sleep, because I was too wiped out to do anything else.

I constantly felt sick, which, combined with an ulcerated mouth and throat that felt like I'd been cut up with razor blades, made eating and drinking near-impossible. I had to use mouthwash every day to stop the ulcers from getting infected. I also took nausea tablets to stop me from throwing up, but sometimes I'd just throw up the nausea tablets.

Oh, and I'll never forget the bone pain, which is a known side effect of doxorubicin. My bones ached 24/7, and the painkillers didn't help much. I felt like I'd been hit by a car.

Week one was hell, and I still had six long months ahead of me. *How does anyone do this?*

Healing Becomes a Full-Time Job

Usually, by the last day of the cycle, the negative effects of the chemo would start to wear off, and I'd try to have a relatively normal day. If I was feeling well enough, I'd get out of the house, maybe go to a café, and make the most of the brief window of vitality I had before going back to the hospital for the next round of treatment.

It was a vicious cycle. Just when I began to feel somewhat normal, they'd shoot me full of chemo drugs again, and I'd be back to feeling like I'd been hit by a car. It was a difficult reality to accept, but I knew I couldn't miss a single chemo session; otherwise, the cancer could spread. I knew I had to be strong and continue the treatment if I was going to beat this thing. That didn't mean I didn't bawl my eyes out whenever I had to leave for the hospital. Mum and Grandad drove me to Peter Mac for every chemo cycle, so I was always leaving Tessa and Fawn behind. Those moments were just as hard as having chemotherapy. I wanted to stay home so badly, just wanted one more hour, one more minute, one more second with Tessa and Fawn before the torture began again. It was even hard looking at Mum and Grandad each time they dropped me off. We would all get upset, but I always pulled myself together and showed them I'd keep fighting, holding my head up high and saying, "Love you."

During this time, my and Tessa's relationship was far from normal. Tessa was basically my full-time carer, and I was so focused on surviving that I didn't always stop to consider what she was going through. It's not like I was being selfish; I'd still tell her I loved her and show my appreciation when I could, but I didn't understand the ripple effects. I didn't understand how my condition would affect the people around me. Tessa was there when I was constantly throwing up in buckets because I didn't have the strength to walk to the toilet or lift my head off the pillow. Many days, I couldn't even stand. She got me water, fed me, tried to make me as comfortable as possible. While I had to dig deep for inner strength, so did she. We were both dealing with a lot.

Grandma frequently came around to massage my feet, whether I was alert or coming in and out of sleep. She tried to keep me as relaxed as possible. Jake often came around in the mornings to check on me and Tessa. One time, he came to get me out of bed, and I looked at him and bawled my eyes out. I didn't want to wake up to the nightmare anymore. The pain, both physical and mental, was unbearable, and I wanted to sleep forever.

All throughout chemotherapy, I felt like I was being pushed beyond what I thought I could handle. It's like driving on a long highway, and the fuel light comes on. You know you've still got a long way to go, but you're almost on empty. *How far until the next servo?* You check how many kilometres your car thinks it can go with what's left in the tank – it doesn't look like you're going to make it. That's how I felt a lot of the time. I was very sick, had no energy, and could barely imagine going another day, let alone another week or month. For every chemo cycle, the fuel light was on, and I never knew if I would make it to the next stop. Thankfully, I *was* able to go the distance, but not without struggle.

Our Origin Story

I met Tessa when I was playing footy at Crib Point Football Club. She played netball, and we trained at the same gym. It was a big club, and we didn't really know each other. Although we'd occasionally say 'hello' and make passing comments, we weren't friends – we'd never had a proper conversation.

I ended up becoming friends with her sister, Leah. Leah was outgoing and talkative, whereas Tessa was quieter and kept to herself, so I didn't get to know her right away. Leah and Tessa trained at the gym together, doing comp prep, while I trained with a couple of my mates, Luke and Mik.

At the time, I was trying to figure out how to make an impact in my footy team. Since starting seniors, I'd been playing full back, even though I'd played in the middle my whole career, so I was looking for any way to improve my game. *How do I get back to the middle?*

One night at the gym, I approached Tessa, asking for help. "How can I get fitter, quicker, stronger?"

"You need to build up your legs. It'll improve your endurance and give you more explosive power." She had a good point. While my upper body was quite strong, I wasn't big on training legs, so my lower body wasn't as powerful as it could've been. Yeah, I was one of those guys who skipped leg day. My bad.

Tessa showed me some leg exercises, and we got talking. I'd got out of a long-term relationship a few months prior, and she was single too. Initially, we were hanging out as friends, training at various gyms together. As it turned out, she was a really down-to-earth person, and we had a good connection. Eventually, on my 21st birthday, we started dating.

Early in our relationship, we took a trip to Thailand, my second home, where I hired a scooter and drove us all around the island and through the jungle as if I were a local.

I knew the place well. On that trip, I got lots of tattoos, and we spent much of the time exploring. I hold those memories close to my heart.

Unfortunately, it wasn't long before my autoimmune issue emerged, so we didn't get to have a normal relationship for long.

The Path to Naturopathy

When I began to experience health issues, Tessa was studying to be an occupational therapist. However, when my autoimmune disease really flared up, we began exploring alternative treatment options, which sent her down a different career path.

The more we learnt, the more Tessa wanted to help people using alternative methods. It was a whole new world of medicine we never knew existed, and we both saw how effective it could be.

Tessa continued studying while I started my business. We eventually saved enough for a house deposit and bought a home at Crib Point. Soon, our dog Fawn joined the family. Although I was experiencing back issues, life was good. Many great things were happening for us. It wasn't long, however, before the autoimmune disease peaked, and I was knocked off my feet, no longer able to so much as walk the dog. All up, we got maybe a year of a normal relationship.

Once I got sick, I was seeing my naturopath frequently, and Tessa attended every session. Sheryl is super-knowledgeable and accomplished in her field, so the opportunity for Tessa to learn from her first-hand was one positive in a sea of negatives. I trusted Sheryl and Tessa with my life, so I was willing to do any protocol they recommended.

Sheryl helped me understand why I had got cancer in the first place and what was happening on a cellular level. I always believed there was a deeper root cause for what was happening to me. Sure, my body had attacked itself and created nasty, cancerous cells – but *why*? If we could understand and address the root cause, there would be no reason for any cancer to return, nor for it to continue to develop.

A Difficult Debt to Repay

Since I got sick, Tessa has been an amazing support. When I couldn't stand, she helped me up. At times, I couldn't stand long enough to shower, so she would guide me to the bath, take my clothes off, and bathe me. She did things like that every day. It takes a really special person to be able to stay so strong in such a tough situation. She basically sacrificed five years of her life to look after me and help me recover. Tessa is an Earth angel, and I wouldn't have been able to survive without her support.

Over the years, I've felt a lot of guilt for being such a burden, and it's something I've had to work through. I'm not forcing Tessa to be here, helping me in my most difficult times. She chooses to be here, and that's what makes her so special. She has put so much effort into getting me where I am today, which is why I have to keep fighting. So many people have sacrificed so much for me, and, to repay them, I'm never giving up. Quitting was never an option.

ZACK'S HEALTH AND WELLBEING TIP

CONSIDER HOLISTIC TREATMENT OPTIONS

While conventional medicine is amazing, it doesn't have all the answers. Sometimes we must search outside the mainstream systems for solutions.

I'm not saying alternative medicine should replace conventional treatment – I chose to embrace both paths to give me the best chance of survival – but they can certainly complement each other. Naturopathy alone can help address many common conditions.[7]

Whatever holistic treatment avenue you choose, the key is to find a knowledgeable practitioner who you trust.

#5

"

I promise you that
what appears today
to be a sacrifice
will prove instead
to be the greatest
investment that you
will ever make.

– GORDON B. HINKLEY

Chapter 6

STRENGTH AND SACRIFICE

Everything's a Gamble

When dealing with a cancer as severe as mine, everything's a risk, from the chemotherapy to the surgery and everything in between. With every step of the treatment process, I was rolling the dice, hoping my number would come up. Sometimes it did, and sometimes it didn't.

As a human being, the unknown is the scariest place to live, but all you can do is keep pushing through the uncertainty and doubt to arrive at the other end. Keeping faith and taking it one day at a time is how I'm here to tell my story today.

Healing Requires Sacrifice

When undergoing aggressive chemotherapy, you'll need to make sacrifices, which can be a tough reality to accept. Due to my autoimmune issue, I'd already given up sport, but I'd managed to hold on to my other passion: carpentry. Even after my initial cancer diagnosis, I was still running my business, and I was still on the tools. At that point, I felt pretty good. I didn't feel like I had cancer; I wasn't coughing up blood, and the only telltale sign that anything was wrong was the lump on my leg.

On workdays, when I needed to go to the hospital for a test or scan, I'd pack up my tools, leave my apprentice with

Dad, who was supervising the site, and drive into the city to Peter Mac, leaving my trailer behind. By the time I returned to the job site, my apprentice would be gone, so I'd just grab my trailer and drive home.

I was supposed to be on crutches to avoid putting weight on the affected leg, as the tumour had eaten into so much of the bone, but I didn't want to stop working. I didn't want to leave that part of my life behind. It wasn't a sacrifice I was ready to make.

However, once I started chemo, I had to be real with myself. There was no way I could work through the after-effects of the treatment. Most days, I could barely walk. So, I explained the situation to my apprentice, who ended up going to work for Dad, and parked my trailer at Tessa's parents' house for the last time. I haven't touched it since.

At that point, it felt like almost everything had been taken away from me. First footy, now carpentry. I'd already sold my motorbike to pay for the faecal transplant; now I'd lost my business and my livelihood. What would be next? The house?

But I couldn't dwell on the sacrifices. If I started thinking life sucked, then life would suck. Yes, I'd made sacrifices, but I hadn't lost everything. I still had Tessa, Fawn, and my beautiful, supportive family. Really, I had more than enough. Soon, however, I was about to have a whole lot more.

Finally, Some Good News!

Almost three months into my treatment, when I was approaching a serious low point mentally and felt like I could no longer handle the pain, the universe threw me a lifeline, another reason to keep fighting.

Tessa was pregnant.

Somehow, in those two weeks of trying before starting chemo, we had succeeded. It felt like a miracle, God's gift, and the news couldn't have come at a better time.

Four months into treatment, I felt utterly depleted. I'd lost 35 kg, couldn't eat, could barely drink, and was stuck in the chemo, flush, rinse, repeat cycle. It was like I was in a washing machine. Ironically, to save my life, they had to take it away from me. During that difficult time, it felt like my unborn son was the only thing keeping me in the fight. The pain was unbearable; I just wanted it to end, one way or another – but I couldn't think like that.

Whenever I felt like giving up, I'd take out the picture of Tessa's 12-week ultrasound to remind myself what I was fighting for. I wanted to meet my son. I wanted to be there for his birth, and long after that. I wanted him to grow up with his dad. He was my drive to keep my head above water and fight each and every day.

Mental Health Nosedive

Even with a new incentive to keep fighting, my mental health continued to deteriorate. I'd been strong so far, but the chemotherapy wasn't just breaking down my body; it was also breaking down my mind. I knew I had to do everything I could to keep fighting. If I ended it, not only would I not get to meet my son, but I'd cause my family more pain, even if I ended mine. I couldn't go down that path. I needed help.

Wasting no time, I signed up for a 12-month mental health program at MyndFit in Mornington. Nick at Mynd-Fit helped me break down what was happening in my life, identifying what I could and couldn't change.

The problem was, while I tried to stay positive throughout treatment, it's not so easy when you're in that type of situation. It wasn't just the pain and the sacrifice; it was also the fact that I couldn't do a lot of the activities that would normally release endorphins. I couldn't run or go to the gym – I couldn't walk at all. During treatment, I switched to crutches, as the tumour had eaten through 80 percent of my bone. If I put too much weight on that leg, it could break, rupture the tumour, and then it'd be a whole different ball game.

Regardless of how much I was suffering, I had to get back into a positive, fighting mindset; otherwise, the battle was lost. The fight wouldn't be over until I said it was. In the end, MyndFit helped me adjust my perspective and strengthen my mental health enough to keep fighting, while my unborn son gave me a reason to fight.

Our Miracle

If you're going through a difficult experience, it's important to have something or someone to fight for, a reason to keep pushing forward. It could be a child, a partner, a pet, whatever gives you strength. I wasn't going to let cancer take me from my family and especially not from my son, soon to be born into this world.

The goal of meeting my son gave me so much strength and hope, and I don't know how far I would've made it without him spurring me on. It's almost as if the universe gave him to us right when we needed him most, when I was close to giving up. He may well have saved my life.

He's very special.

Holding on to My Hair

During treatment, I tried to hang on to my hair as long as possible. While I felt like shit, and probably looked like it too, I didn't want hair loss to mark me as a cancer patient. I wanted to retain some shred of normality, and I refused to shave my head until absolutely necessary. I didn't want cancer to take another thing away from me.

At one point during the holidays, my treatment got pushed back five days, which meant I'd have five extra days of feeling relatively good. So, Tessa and I made the most of it, heading straight to my dad's holiday house in Paynesville to spend some time in nature, with the trees, the birds, and the water, and do a bit of bream fishing.

After spending the last few months in the hospital or stuck on the couch, seeing the beauty of nature again was a wow moment. I'd forgotten what living felt like. I'd forgotten there was a world outside of my own little cocoon of survival. Finally, Tessa and I could spend some quality time together.

One night, we ordered Indian takeaway, and, as I was eating my curry, I noticed something odd in the food. *What's that?* I dug my fingers into the aromatic sauce and retrieved what seemed to be hair. *Where did that come from?* Then some more fell into the bowl. *Oh, shit.* It was *my* hair. I grabbed a tuft from my head, and it came out with no resistance. The battle to keep my hair was over, and I'd lost. I was devastated. Tessa held me and said, "You're still beautiful, the same Zack I fell in love with. Losing your hair doesn't take away the big heart you have."

We ended our little holiday early and drove straight to my grandparents' house. I couldn't stop crying. After everything I'd lost, my hair was gone too. *What next?*

But my despair didn't last long. Grandma used to cut my hair, so she had a set of clippers ready and waiting. She quickly went to work, shaving off what was left of my hair. Next, she brought out a bunch of silly hats, which I tried on, one after another, and we ended up having a really fun night, turning a big low into a massive high.

What started out as a devastating moment became one of my most special memories. I will always hold that night close to my heart. The way Grandma and Grandad made me feel, I'll never forget it. Those moments make or break you. I'm so lucky to have had so much loving support.

Finding Moments of Joy

Because I couldn't walk without crutches, I missed out on walking the dog, even on my good days when I was feeling well enough to leave the house. Tessa would walk Fawn, and

I'd stay home, wishing I was anywhere else. But I was tired of missing out, so I took matters into my own hands.

I went online and found an electric scooter, like what an older person might use when they can no longer walk long distances, and I bought it. My mate Brodie picked it up for me. Now I could join Tessa and Fawn on their walks, get out and taste the fresh air, and listen to the wind in the trees again. I'd often ride my scooter on my old football club's ground, wishing I could have five more minutes on the field or even one more big contest and feel that freedom again.

One group of mates all chipped in and got me a fishing kayak, which changed my life. My happy place is the water. Waking up at the crack of dawn, sitting on the water, watching the sun come up – for me, it's as good as it gets. I would fish all day if I could get away with it. Often, on my good days, I'd hook up the kayak trailer to the scooter and scoot down to the beach, which was about 500 m away from the house. The kayak had a little battery-powered motor, so I didn't even need to paddle. I'd cruise out, find a nice spot, and sit there with my rod for a couple of hours, taking in a bit of life while I could.

In those moments, I felt a sense of freedom I rarely felt anymore. Those small moments of joy kept me going. They reminded me why life was worth living, and why I had to survive.

While there was a lot I couldn't do, I was the most content when I focused on what I could do.

The Next Phase

Although it felt like it would, the six months of chemotherapy didn't last forever. Finally, that stage of treatment was over, and it was time to check the results.

I underwent several tests and scans, many I'd already had before starting chemo, to see how the tumour had responded to the treatment and figure out the best approach for surgery. How much of the bone had the tumour eaten? How much of the bone needed to be removed? Were there any veins in the way? Could we save my leg? There were a lot of questions to answer.

When they performed the radiation scan, I received some startling news – the tumour had shrunk by 95 percent.

"Oh, the chemo worked well," they said.

Little did they know that I'd been sneaking Master's medicinal herbs into the hospital while I was receiving treatment. I'd smuggle the concoction in my bag and drink it during the day. The doctors were against alternative treatments, as they didn't want them interfering with the chemotherapy, but I needed every edge I could get, so I did what I had to do. I truly believe the herbal medicine saved my organs and helped shrink the lump. The doctors would give full credit to the chemo, even though it was never guaranteed to shrink the tumour, mainly just stop it from spreading. If I hadn't taken extra steps to protect myself, I might have died from the overdose of chemo flooding my body. Twenty-percent survival rate, remember? They were hitting me with the hard stuff, and chemotherapy *can* kill.

Unfortunately, the conventional medical system doesn't take a holistic approach to cancer treatment. At least, it didn't with me. Therefore, I had to take my health into my own hands. I spent all my savings and sold what I could to keep up with the alternative treatments. *There's no point having money in my pocket if I'm dead.* It was as simple as that. My mates also set up a GoFundMe to raise money for my treatments, raising almost $20,000, an absolute godsend. I'll be forever grateful to everyone who donated.

On top of everything else, during treatment, I'd often hold my hand over my tumour and visualise it shrinking. The mind is a powerful tool, and focusing on shrinking the lump seemed more useful than sitting there feeling sorry for myself. Whether it worked or not, it certainly didn't hurt.

I'll never know how much of the shrinkage was due to the chemo and how much was due to alternative treatments and lifestyle changes, such as cutting out sugar, but I'd like to think the effort I made had some effect. The doctors, however, only gave credit to the chemo, which was fine.

With the chemotherapy finally over, the next step was surgery.

ZACK'S HEALTH AND WELLBEING TIP

EXPLORE
TRADITIONAL MEDICINE

Many traditional medicines, such as traditional Chinese medicine, have been around for thousands of years – and for good reason. They're often very effective, even if they exist outside of the mainstream in Western cultures.

For me, conventional medicine didn't have everything I was looking for. If I was going to beat cancer, I needed backup. I needed something that would reinforce my body while the chemo tried to destroy it. So, why did Sheryl send me to Master? Because Chinese medicine has been scientifically proven to both increase the efficacy of chemo and radiation therapy while reducing negative side effects.[8] It was exactly what I needed.

Exploring traditional medicine doesn't mean shunning conventional treatment options. It means being open-minded and using everything at your disposal to heal.

#6

Each of us must
confront our own fears,
must come face to face
with them. How we
handle our fears will
determine where we go
with the rest of our lives.

– JUDY BLUME

Chapter 7

LIFE-SAVING SURGERY... AND THE REST

Sense of Betrayal

Even though my tumour had shrunk considerably, my surgeon, Claudia, still wanted to remove the same amount of bone from my shin.

"The scan shows it's only small," I said. "Can't we take less?"

"We have to go off the old scan to ensure we have clear margins," Claudia said. "If we cut into any cancer, it's game over."

I was devastated. Why had I worked so hard to shrink the tumour if they were still going to cut out the same amount of bone? Couldn't they have just cut it out from the start? *Why did I just go through those six months of hell?*

I'd given myself over to the medical system, and now I felt betrayed.

Thankfully, the cancer stayed in the tumour and didn't spread to other parts of my body. However, removing such a big section of bone meant that saving my leg would be difficult. All I could do was roll the dice again and try to have faith.

Best Chance of Survival

Over time, I grew to understand that all of the doctors' and surgeons' recommendations were to give me the best chance of survival. The strong chemo drugs could've killed me, but they were my best chance of survival. The surgery would take more of my shinbone than I was comfortable with, but removing it was my best chance of survival. Essentially, the conventional medical system recommends extreme measures when necessary to increase the odds of survival, no matter the overall cost or collateral damage. The doctors don't want to hold back and risk not doing enough, but sometimes they do push too far.

In my case, by removing so much bone, the surgeons were trying to keep me alive, no matter the impact to my overall lifestyle. The more bone they removed, the less likely it was to properly heal, and the less likely I was to walk again. They'd take my whole leg if they thought it was necessary. Ultimately, the doctors were doing what they thought they had to do to save my life, and I'm grateful, but that didn't make the reality any easier to accept.

At no point was I given any real say in my treatment. It was basically 'accept the process, or you're on your own'. If I hadn't done the chemo, the surgeons would've refused to operate. They didn't want to cut so close to the tumour. I'd done the chemo not only to save my life but also to save my leg, and now I might be sacrificing it anyway.

Do they really have to cut that much? Did the chemo have to be that strong? What if they've made the wrong call? I felt so confused, powerless, and vulnerable. But I'd come this far, so, once again, I surrendered myself to the system and trusted in the process.

Reality Hits

The day before the surgery, I remember standing on the top floor of St Vincent's Hospital, looking out over the city, thinking, *What's going to happen tomorrow? Will they accidentally cut the tumour, causing it to spread through my whole body? Or will the operation be successful? There's a chance I won't wake up at all…*

After months of chemotherapy, I was feeling worn down, to say the least, and maintaining a positive mindset took serious effort. I was running on an empty tank, but I persevered. *Let's get this lump out of me so I can move on with my life. One more battle, Zack. You can do this. Just hold on a little longer.* The surgery didn't just involve removing a chunk of bone from my leg. They'd also be removing muscles, veins, my fibula, and installing the donor bone and a metal plate, knee to ankle, to hold everything in place so my leg could heal. It wasn't exactly a straightforward surgery, and a lot could go wrong.

All up, between the orthopaedic surgeons, plastic surgeons, and everyone assisting, there would be 15 people in the operating room. Yep, the surgery was a big deal.

Before the operation, some of the surgeons came in with an ultrasound machine and a marker, marking where my veins and bones were and how much bone they'd be removing. It's one thing to *say* 22 cm, but to see it marked out like that made the reality hit home.

It was a lot to lose.

Going Under the Knife

Before the operation, the surgeons huddled around my operating bed and explained everything that could go wrong. Basically, I could wake up with my leg in a cage (an Ilizarov apparatus) to hold everything in place, or I could lose my leg completely. Also, the surgery would take 12 to 15 hours, so they'd be working on me practically all day. While the surgeons were confident, I felt like I was rolling the dice yet again, and anything was possible.

Oh, can you guess *when* they chose to explain everything that could go wrong? Right before they put me to sleep. So, my final thoughts before the anaesthetic kicked in were about the worst possible outcomes. Not exactly the best mindset for undergoing life-saving surgery. With thoughts of losing my leg spinning around inside my head, I drifted off to sleep, hoping my number would come up.

When I woke up in the ICU, I immediately asked the nurse, "Is my leg still there?"

"Yeah, love, the surgery went well. Your leg's still there." She was so soothing, so warm; she reminded me of my mum.

"You're like an angel," I said. She smiled. Right then, I felt so much relief. I'd grown so used to hearing bad news that I was always prepared for the worst. This time, however, the news was good.

Once the nurse had checked that I was okay, I was wheeled to a different room to recover, where I slept for an entire day. Because I was on a ketamine drip for the pain, I felt like a zombie. The surgery itself had been hard on my body, and now the drugs were clouding my mind.

Once I was more alert, Claudia visited to explain how the operation had gone. As it turned out, everything had gone well; there were no complications, and all the cancer had been successfully removed. *Yes!* Even though I felt like I'd been hit by a truck, I was thankful for some more good news. With a successful operation behind me, it was time to focus on recovery.

No Shortcuts to Recovery

When I was in hospital, Mum visited every day. She had cut back on her hours at work to try to get me over the line and recovered. She would bring me my Chinese

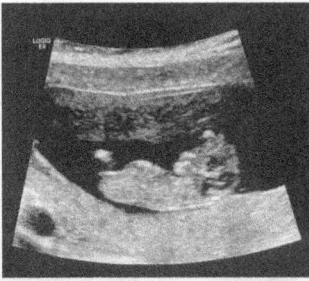

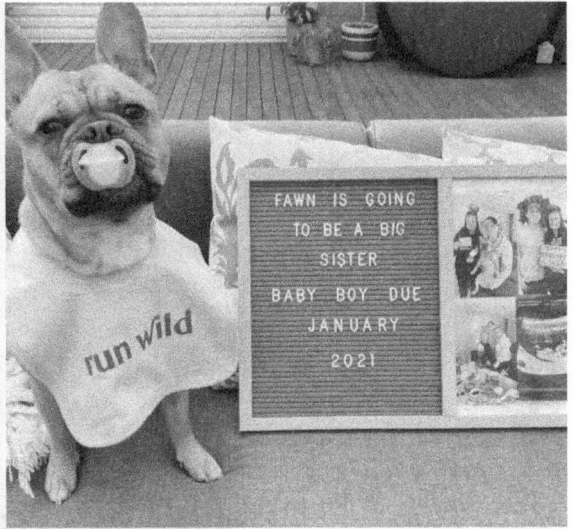

FAWN IS GOING
TO BE A BIG
SISTER
BABY BOY DUE
JANUARY
2021

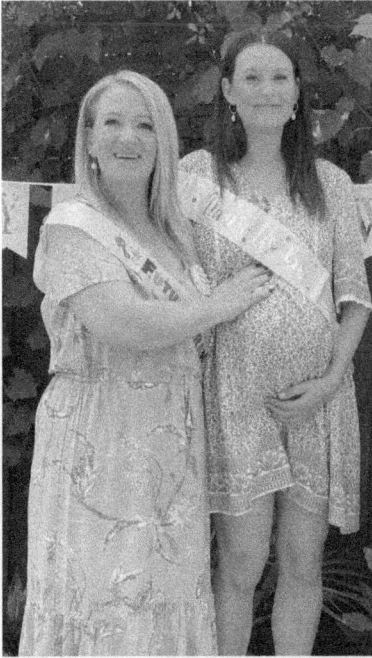

Baby announcement and the ultrasound image that kept Zack in the fight.

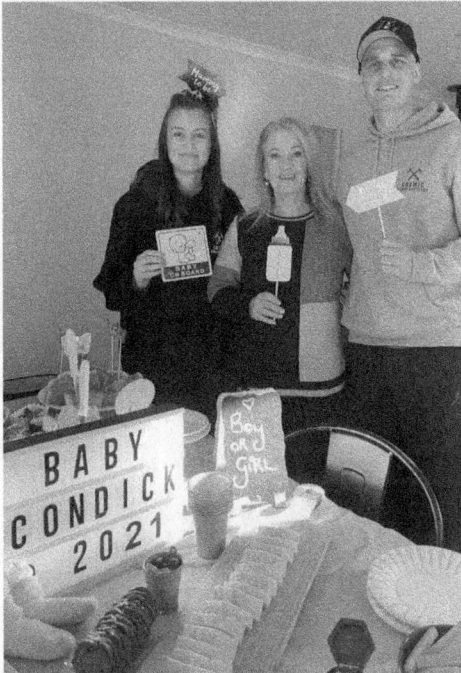

BABY CONDICK 2021

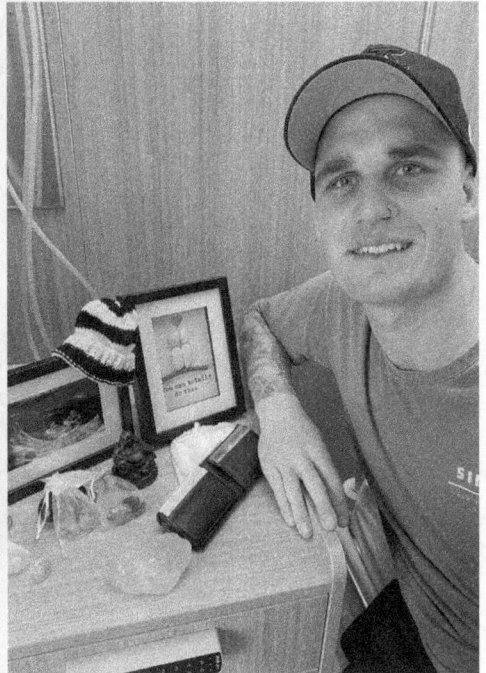

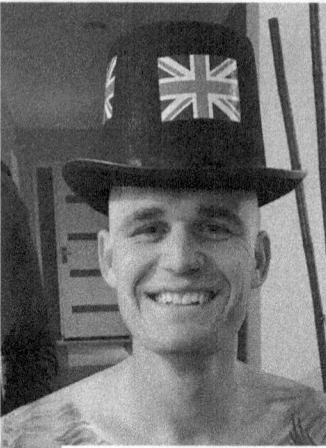

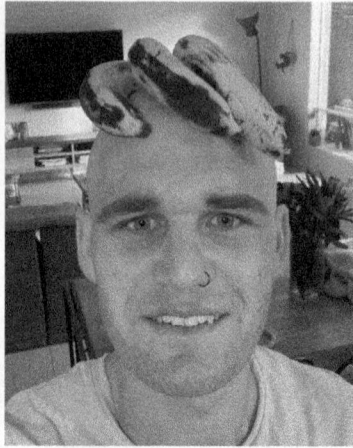

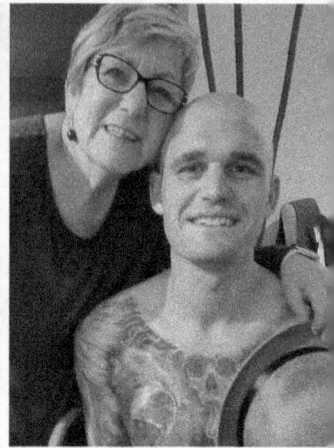

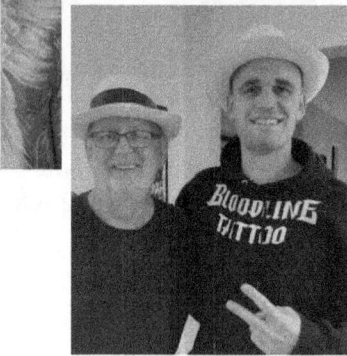

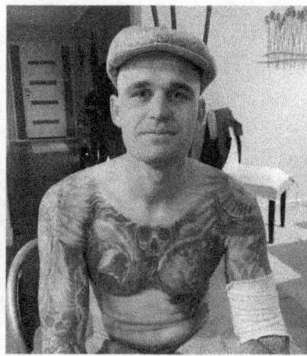

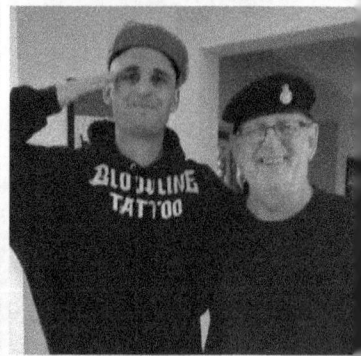

Replacing hair with hats (and other things)
and good times with family and friends.

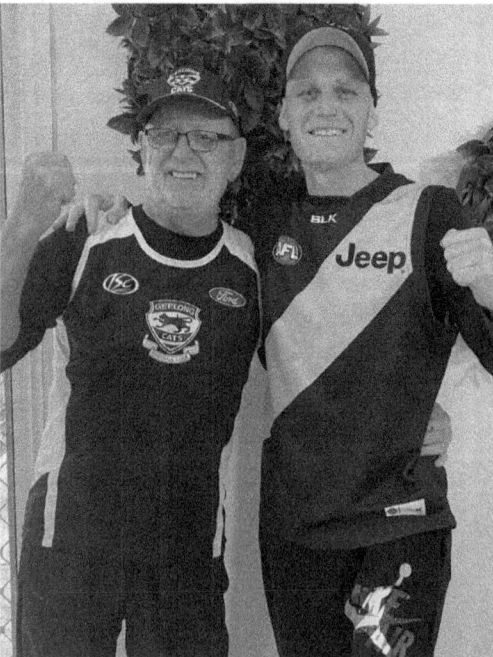

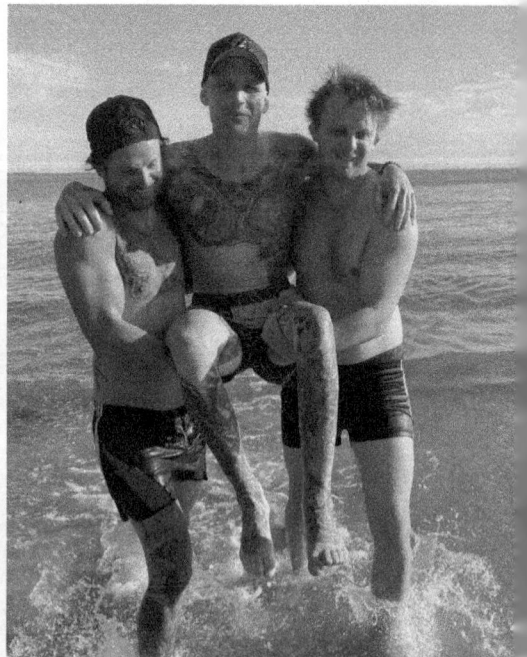

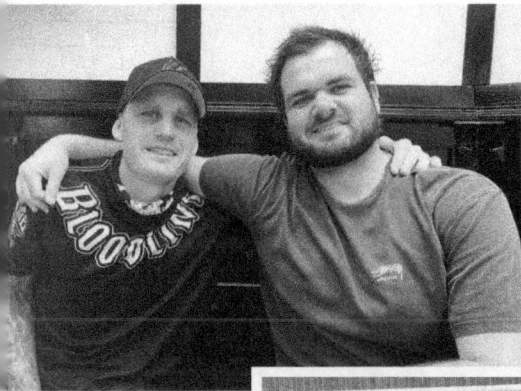

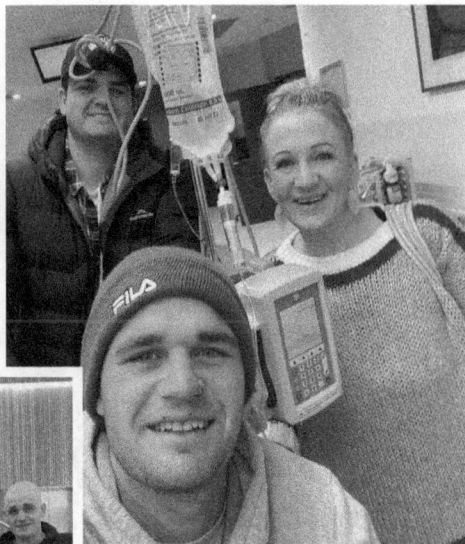

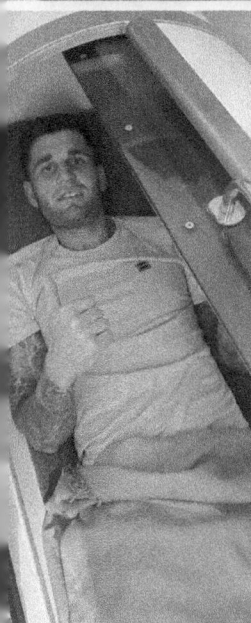

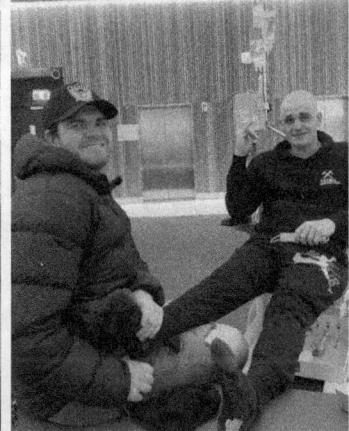

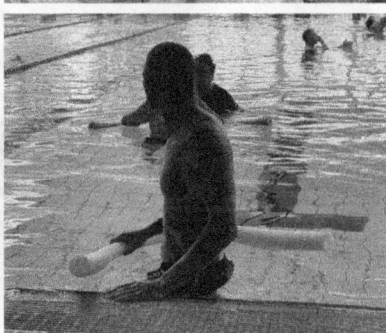

Rehabilitation, recovery, and plenty of fishing.

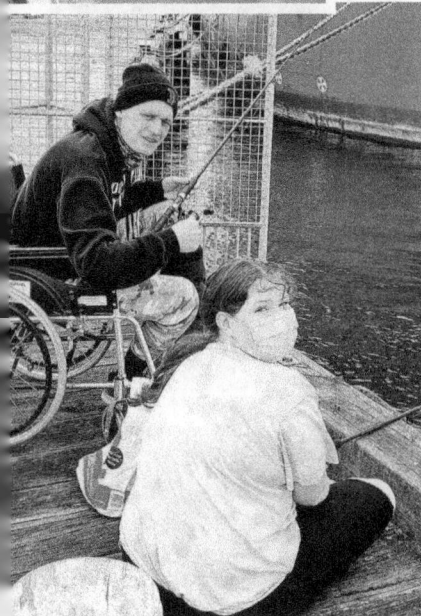

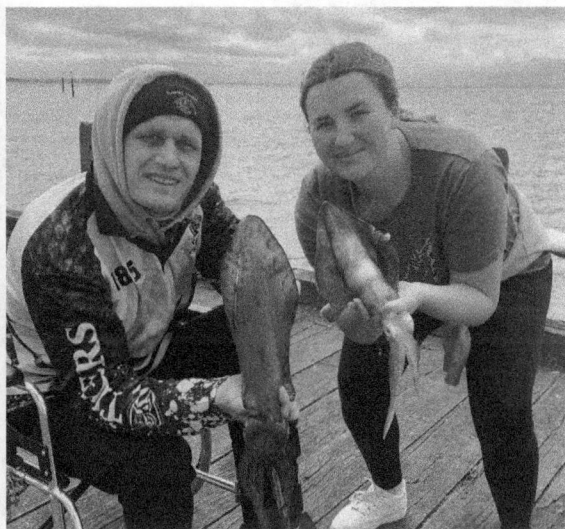

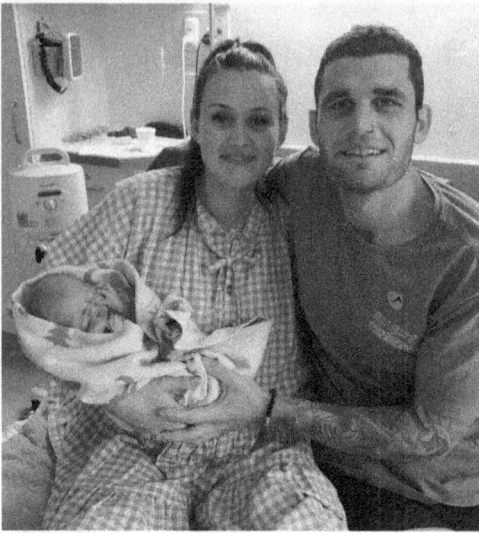

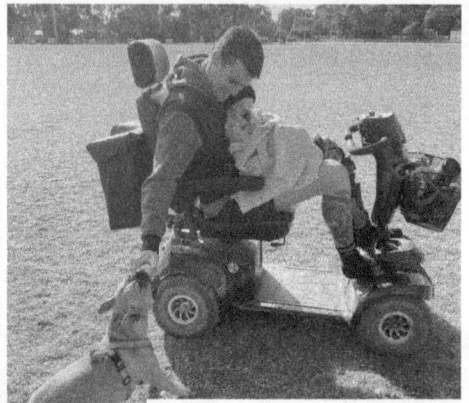

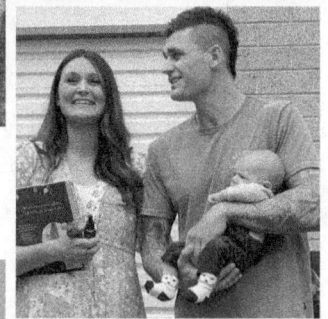

Hunter's birth and name day.

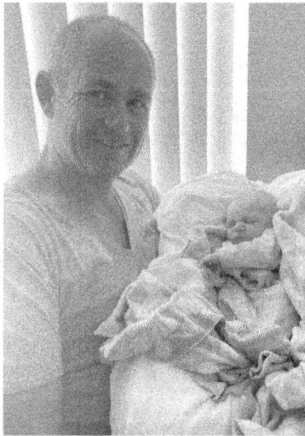

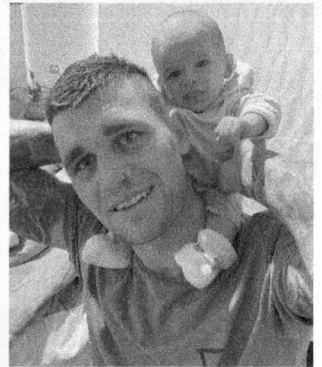

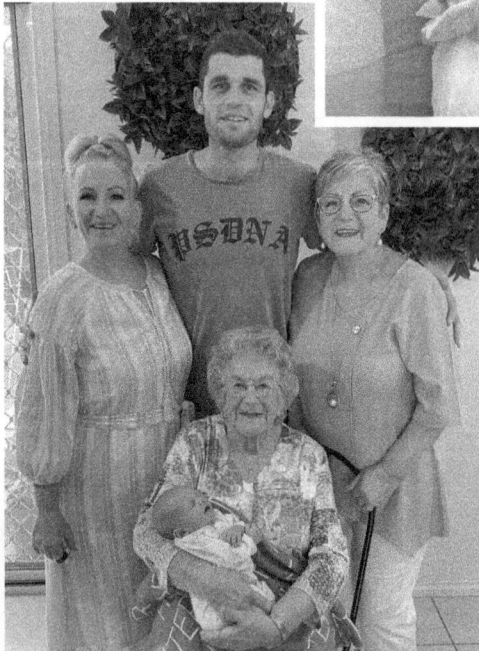

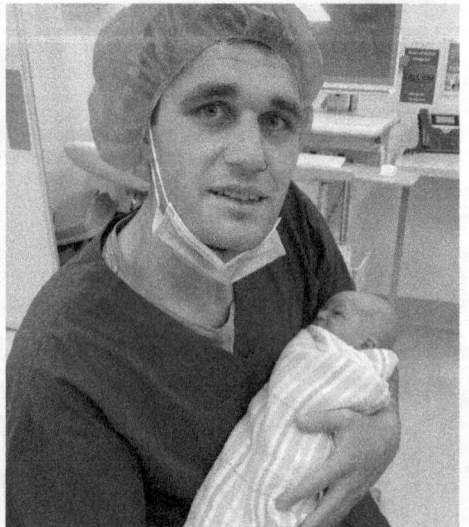

medicine, which I struggled to keep down. I was feeling pretty sick at that point, and, honestly, those healing herbs don't taste great. She also brought me fresh vegetarian food and snacks, so my diet was still on point, and fresh, cold-pressed juices, as it was hard to eat due to the constant agony.

Because I was in a public hospital, I shared a room with another cancer patient, Paul. He'd undergone radiation treatment, not chemo, for a soft tissue cancer, so he'd kept his hair. He had, however, lost his leg, which was confronting to see. I'd never seen anyone with a missing limb before – here he was, right there in the next bed over – and the reality hit home. *It could have been me.* He'd had surgery a week earlier, but his wound wasn't healing, so the doctors were figuring out what to do next. There was talk of another surgery. I, however, was in the clear, for now at least, and was ready to start physiotherapy.

"All right, Zack," the physio said, "I want to see you try and get to the toilet."

I was sore as hell – I'd just had almost my entire shinbone cut out, not to mention my entire fibula – but I forced myself to sit up and slid off the bed. It was the first time since waking up that my legs hadn't been elevated. It was the first time they'd touched the ground. As the blood rushed to my feet, the pain was excruciating. It felt like someone was hacking at my leg with a samurai sword. Along with the bone, they'd cut out half of my inner calf where the tumour had been. Blinding pain thumped through my leg, and I almost blacked out.

All right, I thought, *better make this quick.* The toilet was only a couple metres away, but it felt like a mile. Using two crutches, with blood bags hanging off me to continuously drain excess blood that was pooling in my leg, I laboured towards the toilet. Immediately feeling out of breath, I thought I was going to collapse. Finally, I made it to the toilet and dropped down hard onto the seat. It wasn't a graceful landing at all, but I'd made it. However, the victory was short-lived. Before I knew what was happening, I'd thrown up all over myself from the pain. My legs throbbed; my head throbbed, and I was struggling to breathe. *Crutching a couple metres to the toilet nearly killed me. How am I going to get through the next few months?* Clearly, the road to recovery was going to be rough, and the light at the end of the tunnel looked very far away.

A Powerful Bond

Recovering in hospital, I spent most of my days lying in bed. By this point, the COVID pandemic had kicked off, which meant only Mum was allowed to visit. She couldn't be there for every second of the day, so I spent a lot of time talking with Paul. When we couldn't sleep due to the pain, we'd watch morning fishing shows and chat. We'd talk about what we'd been through and what we wanted for the future – marriage, kids, career, everything. Paul wanted to be a doctor, and I reassured him that he didn't need two legs for that. "Don't let cancer wreck your dream career," I said. "We'll get you a good wheelchair." I showed him the ultrasound picture of my unborn son, which I always kept with me, explaining that I had a kid on the way. He didn't have any kids, but he loved his dog. He had a photo of him at the end of his bed. All he wanted to do was go home and hug that dog. When you've been through hell and faced death, all materialism goes out the window, and you just want more time with the people you love. For most of us, it's a complete perspective shift.

Due to the pandemic, Paul's family wasn't allowed to visit, so Mum brought in food and drinks for him whenever she visited. Every day, we supported each other, building each other up as much as we could, giving each other the strength to fight another day. We especially supported each other through our physio sessions, which were painful and exhausting. We understood what each other was going through, and we built a friendship, a powerful bond, so I felt a lot of guilt when I had to leave him behind.

After two weeks in hospital, I was given the all clear to go home. My wound wasn't bleeding, and I could get around on crutches. However, the excruciating pain hadn't faded at all. I was still living in agony. The solution? "Here are some painkillers, go home and rest."

During my two weeks in hospital, Paul had another surgery because his wound refused to heal, so he was going through some shit. I felt like I was leaving a soldier behind. After we said our goodbyes, he had to watch me walk out of there with my mum, while he was stuck in the hospital for the foreseeable future. To soften the blow, Mum helped Paul's girlfriend get an exemption to come and visit him for the day. He was so thankful for that and everything else Mum did for him.

After I left hospital, Paul and I kept in touch. When we were both feeling better, we planned to catch up. We even discussed being at each other's weddings. We couldn't wait to meet up and see how well we'd recovered and what we were doing with our new lives. First things first though – I needed to focus on my recovery.

Relentless Recovery Protocol

The intense pain lasted for over a month, and I was starting to think I'd never be pain-free again. Because I had no prior experience with surgery, I didn't know exactly what I was in for recovery wise, and the constant agony, with seemingly no progress, was demoralising. *Will I ever walk again?* With the pain and painkillers messing with my head, I couldn't help but question my recovery.

I felt constantly exhausted, and some days I could barely get from the bed to the couch. Not only did Tessa have to care for me through chemo, but now she was back in the carer's role, helping me get around the house. Often, I couldn't even get out of bed. All I could do was lie there on my back, dosed up on painkillers, hoping for the pain to end. It was a tough recovery. Tessa often had to bring me a bottle to pee in. That's how sore I was. I didn't want to move an inch and set off even worse pain.

Three months, they said, and I'd be off crutches and starting to walk again. *Three months? I can handle that.* At least I had a rough timeline for when I'd be back on my feet. Then came the bad news.

"We need to get you back into chemotherapy, but we also need to give you some time to heal."

"Okay, when do I start?"

"Two weeks."

"Two weeks?" Fucking hell. I had just gone through six months of chemo, serious surgery, hadn't recovered, was still in severe pain, and they wanted me to jump right back into chemo. They had to be joking, right?

Apparently, if I left it too long, the cancer could return and spread. 'Mop-up treatment', they called it. But what about my leg? Wouldn't the chemo impede the healing process? But the doctors knew best, and they were adamant that I needed to resume chemotherapy as soon as possible.

At this point, my fuel gauge was in the red zone. Six months of gruelling chemotherapy, a 15-hour surgery, now more chemo – I was almost empty. I looked up at the sky and pleaded with the universe. "Please help me make it through this mop-up treatment. I want to meet my unborn son. I want it more than anything… please." I hoped someone was listening.

Bitten Again

About a month after surgery, I was back on chemo. I already felt like crap, so, in my mind, it was the last thing I needed. During this time, I kept taking my herbal medicines and going to Master for Qigong healings, this time focusing on healing my leg. As expected, the chemo knocked me around a lot, but I was pushing through, knowing that the end was near. *I can get through this,* I thought. *I did it before, I'll do it again.*

Then I got bitten by a spider.

We'd just had a woodfire heater installed, so I'm guessing the spider came off the wood. Normally, a spider bite wouldn't be a big deal, but the chemotherapy had made me neutropenic, lowering my white blood cell levels. Basically, my body struggled to fight off infection – bad news when you've been bitten by a spider.

The next day, I woke up with a lump on my hand. Before long, I got hit with a massive fever – almost 40°C – and I was worried I'd go into a coma. Even so, I didn't want to get medical care. I didn't want to spend the rest of the week in hospital for a spider bite only to go into Peter Mac for chemo the next week. I had never liked hospitals, and, at that point, I was done. I just wanted to stay at home until my next round of treatment. My stubbornness almost got me killed.

Even though I had two jumpers on and was sitting by the fire in a wheelchair, I was still shivering – I couldn't get warm. Eventually, I lost feeling in my arms, and Mum announced she was calling an ambulance. At that point, I couldn't argue.

When the ambulance arrived, the paramedics checked me over, gave me something to help the fever, and recommended that I go with them to hospital for monitoring and fluids. As Jake was wheeling me towards the front door, I didn't even have the strength to hold my head up, and I threw up all over myself. After getting cleaned up, I was loaded into the ambulance. When I looked back at Tessa, I cried, once again not wanting to leave her for the hospital. Unfortunately, I had no choice but to let them take me.

ZACK'S HEALTH AND WELLBEING TIP

PRACTISE MEDITATION

When I was experiencing the worst of my pain and anxiety, meditation helped me stay grounded. I could've easily let my thoughts spiral and become stuck in a negative mindset, but, over time, I learnt to better control my thinking and, for the most part, maintain a positive outlook. Hey, it wasn't always easy, but, for me, it was necessary.

Meditation has several proven benefits, including stress, anxiety, and depression reduction, reduced physical and psychological pain, and decreased blood pressure.[9] Considering what I was going through with chemo and recovery, it's no wonder meditation was so helpful.

There are many different types of meditation practices out there, so, if you're interested in giving it a go, find one that works for you and make it a regular part of your routine.

#7

"

Out of suffering have emerged the strongest souls; the most massive characters are seared with scars.

– KAHLIL GIBRAN

Chapter 8

PEAKS AND VALLEYS

Like I Had the Plague

When I was admitted to Frankston Hospital with a spider bite, I had no idea what I was walking, or being wheeled, into. This happened in September 2020, when the COVID pandemic was still in full force. During that time, anyone presenting COVID symptoms, like a fever for instance, was treated like they had the plague. The hospital was in a state of pure panic.

Even though I showed them the spider bite and tried to explain my medical history and that I was neutropenic from chemotherapy, the doctors didn't want to believe me. To them, I was a COVID case until proven otherwise, and I was put in a room by myself, isolated from the outside world. No one wanted to come near me.

Eventually, Mum managed to get into the hospital, bringing me some health foods and cold-pressed juices, which the staff promptly lost or threw away. I was stuck in a wheelchair, hooked up to an IV fluid drip, and I couldn't even get to the toilet by myself. My leg was still recovering from surgery, so I was on two crutches. With an IV pole connected to me, how did they expect me to get to the toilet? Although I kept clicking the buzzer, calling for help, no one came for a long time, and I almost shat myself. Due to the fluid drip, I needed to go to the toilet a lot, and constantly getting up was almost too painful to bear. I felt like I was overheating, but there wasn't much I could do. I just sat there in my jocks, with cold flannels and ice, trying to cool my body down. I was so worried about going into a coma that I couldn't sleep at all. I just kept getting fresh ice and changing my flannel over and over. I felt like I was living in hell.

A Soul-Crushing Experience

After everything I'd been through, that time in the hospital was the closest I got to giving up. First the autoimmune disease, then the cancer diagnosis, then the chemo, then the surgery, then more chemo, and now a spider bite had almost taken me out.

I can't take much more of this.

I ended up staying in hospital for a week, taking a heavy dose of antibiotics to clear the infection. It was the scariest week of my life. I'd sit there, looking out the window, not caring about what was happening around me, not caring about what was happening *to* me. Grandma came in to visit and rub my feet, and I didn't care that she was there. Clearly, something was wrong. It felt like my soul had left my body.

Mum realised what was happening and demanded that I be discharged immediately. At the time, she worked at Frankston Hospital but had cut her shifts right back to help care for me. She talked to the right people and got me released, with a tank of antibiotics in a fanny-pack-like device hooked up to my PICC line.

The spider bite had almost killed me. It was time to draw the line.

Taking Back Control

Up until that point, I'd done everything the doctors had asked me to do. I did the chemo; I let them take my shinbone, and I went back for more chemotherapy – but enough was enough.

At the end of the day, no one really knows what's going to happen, and I knew it was time to take my health back into my own hands.

My latest scans hadn't shown any cancer in my body, so the mop-up treatment was just a precaution. Yes, it was highly recommended, but it could also be causing unnecessary harm. I was doing the chemotherapy to save my life, but it felt more like it was taking it. I'd reached my limit, and I had to do what I felt was right for me.

While I figured out exactly what to do, I ignored the calls from Peter Mac and didn't go in for any more chemo treatments. I needed space to clear my head. I needed my soul back. Of course, everyone was worried about me, but I had to get myself out of that negative thought spiral.

To help build myself back up mentally, I took another trip to Paynesville with Tessa and Jake, where I did some fishing and spent time near the water. I wanted to start bringing the activities I enjoyed back into my life so I could feel like I was living again. As I began to feel more like myself, I knew what I had to do.

Eventually, my oncologist got hold of Mum, and she explained my decision. I'd be stopping chemo for good.

"We're worried about his wellbeing," Mum said. "The chemo's killing his body. He's disintegrating. He's lost thirty-five kilos, and he can't move. A spider bite nearly killed him. The scan shows no remaining cancer, so he's stopping the treatment. We honestly don't know if he'd make it through another round."

I went to Peter Mac for a meeting, and, of course, the doctors tried to persuade me to continue with the treatment, but I couldn't handle another three months of chemotherapy. My mind couldn't take it, and I don't think my body could either. Besides, at that stage of my recovery, I felt like I would do better on Master's herbs and Sheryl's naturopathic protocols.

Finally, I felt like I had a say, and I chose to stop chemotherapy, rolling the dice again and having faith that holistic medicine would get me through.

They Thought I Was Insane

Mum was so supportive of my decision. She knew everything I'd been through, and she understood all the extra work I'd been doing to support my health, so she backed me completely.

The doctors thought I was crazy for stopping chemo, so they sent me to a counsellor to check my mental state.

"Can you live with yourself if you stop treatment early and the cancer comes back?" the counsellor asked.

"I can live with knowing that I stopped something I thought was going to kill me," I said. "I can't do it anymore."

"All right, no worries."

And that was that. I signed some forms and agreed to come back for scans every three months to make sure the cancer hadn't returned. I got my PICC line taken out that day and went home, no longer a cancer patient but a cancer survivor.

A Devastating Phone Call

On 7 October 2020, I got a phone call that hit me like a wrecking ball. My best mate Brodie's partner Georgia was on the other end, crying. *Oh, no.* "What happened?" I asked. "Is Brodie okay?"

I never wanted anyone close to me to feel or endure the pain and suffering I experienced during my battle with cancer. I never wanted anyone to face death like I had. I asked the universe to keep my family and friends healthy and happy, saying I would take the hit for everyone if necessary. Apparently, my proposal was rejected.

"It's Mav," she said. Mav was their newborn son.

"What's wrong with Mav? Is he okay?"

"He's been rushed to the Royal Children's Hospital. He… they said he's got leukemia."

No… no, no, no, no, no. I couldn't utter a word in response. I dropped the phone and bawled my eyes out. It felt like my heart had been ripped out. Brodie and Georgia had supported me all throughout my cancer battle, and now they had their own battle to fight. Without missing a beat, Tessa and I provided our full support, helping in any and every way we could.

Thankfully, this story has a happy ending. After undergoing gruelling chemotherapy for several years, Mav is now cancer-free and living a normal childhood.

Getting the Old Zack Back

Over time, the old Zack started to come back. While I still couldn't get around without crutches, I no longer had the burden of chemotherapy weighing me down. I was cancer-free and ready to tackle the next set of challenges.

After deciding to quit chemo, I felt more in control of my life, and I continued the alternative treatments, building my body back up with Master's medicine and other nutritious foods. I did everything in my power to help my leg heal. I wanted to be in the best state possible, both physically and mentally, when my son arrived.

Everything seemed to be going well until...

I Lost a Friend

In November of 2020, Paul passed away. Before his passing, he sent me a text message. He explained what an impact Mum and I had on his life and how grateful he was to have known us. He also told me to kick the cancer's arse and walk again – to do it for him. Then he said he was going into palliative care. When the message came through, I was in the car with Mum, and I broke down crying. I was devastated.

I tried to get to Geelong, where he was in care, to see him, but I was barely mobile, relying on other people to get me around, and it was a two-hour drive. Although I couldn't get there right away, I did plan to go on the weekend to say my final goodbyes, but I was too late. He died only two days after he sent that message. His partner texted me off his phone, saying, *Paul's gone*. Just like that.

Paul's death hit hard. When you're facing major health issues and possible death, it's hard to explain to people what you're going through. While they try to understand, if they haven't experienced it themselves, they don't fully get it. In Paul, I found someone I could finally relate to. Now, he was gone. His death also drove home the reality that cancer can come back and kill us at any time. It has to be taken seriously. I was so grateful I'd done all the alternative therapies on top of the conventional treatments. Many, like Paul, only take the conventional route, and I can't help but wonder if more people would have lived if they'd supported their bodies better throughout treatment.

In Paul's case, his cancer had returned and gone to his chest. There was nothing they could do.

A New Light in My Life

In January 2021, Hunter was born. Right before his birth, my hair grew back. Weirdly, I'd always had straight hair, but it grew back wavy with blonde streaks through it. So, in my first photos with Hunter, I had a full head of hair. It's nice to look back on those pictures and see me looking relatively healthy, with my hair and eyebrows intact. If it had been a month earlier, I would've looked completely different. I didn't want to look like a cancer patient in my first photo holding my son.

When Hunter was born, I sent a message to Paul's phone with a picture of me holding my son. *I'm going to be a dad for both of us. I'm going to beat this, and I'm going to walk again.* Although he was no longer here to receive the message, it felt good to send it to him anyway.

Because I was still on crutches, having a newborn baby was challenging to say the least. Tessa had to have an emergency C-section, which meant she couldn't bend over or do any heavy lifting for six weeks. I'll admit, when the placenta ruptured and they rushed her to surgery, it triggered a lot of emotions. *Surely, this isn't happening...* I'd taken so many hits over the past few years that it didn't seem out of the realm of possibility that the birth would go wrong too. Thankfully, the procedure went well, and Hunter was born a healthy, happy boy.

A Real Team Effort

Being a carpenter, if I'd been able to, I would've done all the work to get Hunter's room ready. Because I couldn't lift or walk, we had to improvise. I explained to Tessa what to do, and she did the work. It wasn't the ideal solution, but it worked out in the end. At that point, we'd got used to things being less than ideal.

The challenges didn't stop there.

Because neither of us could get up to Hunter in the night – I couldn't put weight on my leg, and Tessa couldn't lift – he slept in our bed between us in his bassinet so he was always close by. Once again, it wasn't the ideal solution, but it mostly worked.

While we managed to solve most problems, we couldn't do it all alone, and Mum, Jake, my sister Olivia, Grandma, and Grandad pitched in a lot. It was a real team effort, and they all helped in their own ways. Mum cooked, did the washing and house cleaning, and took me on coffee dates. Jake and Olivia helped with Hunter and were great emotional support. Grandma did all the house stuff with Mum and frequently gave me foot and leg massages to relieve the swelling and pain. When I lost my hair, she also gave me daily head massages, as the headaches from the chemo were unbearable. Grandad, in his 70s, mowed our lawns and put our bins out every week. He also attended every one of my medical appointments. He has been with me every step of the way. Tessa's parents, Julie and Garry, also helped out a lot, dropping off meals every night for a year and helping to pay the bills, which relieved some of the financial pressure. I had an amazing team around me and if it wasn't for them, I wouldn't be here to tell my story now.

After so much negativity in our lives, Hunter was a true blessing. Suddenly, we were focused on something positive, and it filled us all with hope. Before, most conversations with friends or family would start with, "How's the leg?"

Now it's, "How's Hunter?" After losing so much, I'd finally gained something beautiful and amazing. I was a dad! It was a welcome change for us all, and I'm so glad I kept fighting and survived to be in Hunter's life.

A Beautiful Soul

Due to my condition – not being able to walk – I was fighting to get support from the NDIS (National Disability Insurance Scheme), and it was a fight I was losing. I had to prove that I had a permanent impairment, and no one could say for sure whether my current condition would be permanent or not. We just didn't know.

Note: I did eventually get my NDIS application approved after 2.5 years, but not without a big fight. It was an exhausting process, but I'm grateful for the support I now receive. It makes my life so much easier. It allows me to concentrate on my healing and rehab regime so I can give my leg the best chance of healing. I have Jane and Michelle who cook and clean each week so I can pursue my dream of going to the city to train for the para rowing team and try to make the Paralympics. Without these beautiful ladies, I couldn't put in the extra time at the pool and gym and see my physios, giving my leg every chance to heal.

Because I had no NDIS support and no income, Imelda, a massage therapist and all-round amazing lady, would come over and massage my feet at night. She was a godsend. I've known Imelda since I was 18. She used to massage me when I played footy, and she quickly became family. When I was really struggling with my health, she'd pray for me, and she asked the church to light a candle when I had my surgery. After my surgery, she knew how much pain I was in, so she frequently made time for me, no matter how busy she was. Even when I was in so much pain that I couldn't move off the couch, she would drive to my house and massage me. She always made me feel good, more hopeful, more alive. She's a beautiful soul, and her visits helped keep me afloat when I was drowning in pain and uncertainty. Her wisdom and positivity lit up my soul and gave me hope.

Here We Go Again...

In April 2021, I learnt that the operation hadn't been a complete success after all. While some healing had taken place–X-rays showed some fogginess between the top and bottom joins – there wasn't a strong connection. If the donor bone didn't take, it would need to be removed. Did the chemotherapy affect the healing process? I can't know for sure, but I do wonder.

So, what was the solution?

My surgeon, Claudia, suggested using bone grafts to fertilise the joins and hopefully prompt them to heal. The plan was to take a chunk of bone from my heel, turn it into a paste – 'bonecrete' – and insert it between the joins. I agreed to the procedure and found myself back in the same ward at St Vincent's where I'd met Paul, which was tough to handle. Staring out the same window that Paul and I had looked out each day triggered me a lot. It was very traumatic. My emotions overwhelmed me. I became abrupt with people, rude, standoffish. I wasn't myself.

After the operation, which went well, I was on heavy pain-killers. They clouded my thinking, and I don't remember much of my time in the hospital. I just knew I wanted to get home, be in my own space, and get off the medication.

Once again, I was recovering from surgery, but at least this time I didn't have chemo interfering with the healing process. In a way, it was back to square one – wheelchair, crutches, several months of waiting for the bone to heal before I could start rehab again. I'd been here before. With a relatively healthy body, I hoped the operation would be my last and I'd be walking unassisted in a few short months – that was the plan. You've probably realised by now that few things in my life ever go to plan.

ZACK'S HEALTH AND WELLBEING TIP

TAKE THE (COLD) PLUNGE

As part of my routine and recovery, I do a cold plunge every single day. I've been doing it for a while, and it never gets easier. I always want to back out. However, by regularly taking the plunge, I've maintained, and perhaps even further developed, my mental toughness. Hey, it's not easy forcing yourself to sit in ice-cold water for minutes on end. Don't believe me? Try it.

Aside from toughening us up, what other benefits do cold plunges, or ice baths, provide? Potential benefits include reduced inflammation, improved mood and cognition, and a more balanced nervous system.[10] Personally, I've experienced all these and more. I wouldn't be putting myself through it every day if I wasn't seeing some benefits. With that said, I'm well aware that ice baths aren't for everyone, and a cold shower might be more appropriate for some. Do whatever works for you.

If you're considering taking the plunge, you should first consult with a medical professional to discuss potential risks.

#8

"

I can be changed
by what happens
to me. But I refuse
to be reduced by it.

– MAYA ANGELOU

Chapter 9

REBUILDING A SHATTERED LIFE

Searching for Normalcy

After my second surgery, I continued to put all my effort into healing and rehabilitation. I continued with the Chinese medicine, cooking up herbs every day, and, over time, I was putting more and more weight on my leg, eventually getting down to one crutch and 60–80 percent weight bearing.

All throughout my treatment and recovery, I searched for new ways to heal myself more effectively. For example, after my second surgery, I began using a hyperbaric chamber, which, if you're unfamiliar with the treatment, is a form of oxygen therapy. Basically, you lie in a pressurised chamber where the air pressure is higher than outside, which helps your body get more oxygen to the tissue, enhancing the healing process.

I also got a set of Normatec compression boots, which can help with recovery. On top of that, I researched ways to heal bone and got an EXOGEN bone healing machine, which uses ultrasound to stimulate bone growth. I also rubbed comfrey cream into my leg morning and night. Comfrey, aka 'knitbone', has been used to heal tissue and bone for centuries. Most days, I also drank hydrogen water – water with added hydrogen – for general health.

Essentially, I left no stone unturned. All the little things I did to support my body's healing had the potential to add up to something big. It was my leg on the line, and I was willing to do everything possible to save it.

Progress was slow, but I was seeing results, and I could almost imagine a time when I'd be able to walk again. It felt like I had a fresh start at my fingertips, and I was ready to move on with my life.

With my recovery progressing, I felt more like myself, but something was missing. I wasn't used to sitting around. I'd been working since before I left school, and I wanted a bit of normality back in my life. Plus, my savings and GoFundMe money had run out, so I needed an income to pay for my house and medicine. But what could I do? With only one good leg, carpentry wasn't an option. I didn't want to sit in an office doing telemarketing calls or anything like that. I wanted to be outside in the fresh air.

I ended up buying an old tip truck and did some small jobs for people. During this time, I called up a lot of businesses, looking for stable work, but all I received was knockback after knockback. In my current state, and perhaps due to work safety concerns, no one wanted to touch me.

Eventually, I got in touch with Michael, a landscaper who lived next door to a house Dad was building. I'd been playing around on Dad's excavator, which I didn't need my legs to operate, and got pretty competent with it. I offered to operate an excavator and Posi-Track for Michael in his landscaping business, and he agreed to take me on. Finally, someone saw past the crutches and gave me the normality I needed. What an awesome guy to give me a crack, getting me back working and giving me an opportunity to get my life back. I wouldn't let him down. I would show him I was worthy and could still be as efficient as a fully abled worker. I can't thank him enough for giving me an opportunity.

Being in a work environment, being around people again, and making friends had a positive impact on my mental health. Each shift, I'd throw my crutches up into the excavator, hop in, and dig all day. Because I was also doing pool rehab, I only worked a couple of days a week, but it was a good balance. As well as the mental health benefits, it was good to have some money coming in so I could keep up with my alternative treatments. I didn't want to stop my Chinese herbs, because they were preventing the cancer from coming back, and they were supporting my bones to heal.

Nowadays, all the alternative therapies and supplements I use are a part of a lifestyle aimed at prevention, not cure. Maybe me getting sick had a purpose. Perhaps it was to give me the knowledge and experience to show others how to look after themselves, to fight even the seemingly unwinnable battles, and to enjoy the simple things in life.

When I was digging, Michael never rushed me, never cracked the whip; he just encouraged me to do the work in my own time. On one job, we did an entire soccer field, and accomplishing something so big made me feel human again. After everything I'd been through, I'd lost a lot of confidence, and being able to work again was an important part of my recovery. In this, Michael's support was invaluable. He gave me a shot when no one else would. I'll never forget his generosity and the authentic support he gave me each day.

Never Pass on a Good Opportunity

I've found that if you want something in life, you have to keep pushing for it. I got knocked back so many times looking for work that I could've just given up and assumed no one would ever hire me. After all, it's not very often you see a guy on crutches getting around a job site.

Ultimately, I had to trust the process and know that, if I kept working for it, I'd eventually get what I needed. The universe has a funny way of giving us just what we need at the right time. Suddenly, everything lined up, with Dad working next to a guy who needed soil moved. When those opportunities appear, it's important to grab hold of them. You can't expect the universe to do all the work. You must act too.

My Stubborn Leg

Several months after my second surgery, while I'd got down to one crutch and could put some weight on my leg, I still couldn't walk unassisted. Unfortunately, scans showed that my body hadn't accepted the grafted bone and had instead absorbed it. Absorption was always a possibility, but the gamble was worth it. This time, however, I'd rolled the dice, and my number hadn't come up – at least not yet.

Because the donor bone wasn't alive, healing was ten times harder. The body realised the bone was foreign, so I needed to do everything in my power to give my leg the best chance of healing, which included continuing with my holistic therapies.

When there's so much uncertainty, so much unknown, scan days can be very traumatic. For me, it's all nerves, anticipation, hope, and dread, all swirling around inside my head. *What if the cancer has come back? What if my leg isn't healing? What if there's some new problem we never saw coming?* After each scan, I generally spend the next couple of weeks trying to shake off the lingering anxiety. It always sticks with me for a while afterwards. Of course, I do try to remain positive, but, after everything that has happened, I've learnt to hope for the best but prepare for the worst. Hey, I've got to be realistic. Sometimes the news isn't good.

The next course of action was to try to stimulate growth by putting more weight on the leg. If we could irritate the joins enough for my body to notice the gap, it would promote the healing process. However, as much as we tried to make the bone grow, it was too stubborn, and healing had essentially stalled.

So, what was the solution? More surgery, this time starting from scratch to completely reconstruct the leg. Oh, but it gets worse. They couldn't reuse the fibula they'd placed alongside the donor bone. It had to be discarded, and they'd need to replace it with the fibula from my good leg. Apparently, I'd still be able to walk without it – the surgeons said it was like a spare tyre – but that leg would never be as strong and stable again.

Once again, I had a tough decision to make.

Choosing the Best of the Bad

If I went ahead with the proposed surgery, option one, they'd need to take everything out of my leg – the donor bone, the fibula, and the metal plates that were holding everything in place, essentially leaving me empty. It would be another massive surgery, another 15-hour reconstruction, opening up two legs at the same time, knee to ankle.

The second option was a below-knee amputation – cut off the bottom half of the leg and use a prosthetic for the rest of my life. Not exactly ideal.

The third option was to travel to Italy and have the same surgery but with a donor bone with tissue and veins still attached so my body wouldn't see it was foreign. In Australia, any bones that go into the bone bank need to be chemically cleaned so no tissue remains, reducing the risk of infection. The problem is, the bone basically becomes a hollow, albeit strong, piece of timber. It's not alive, and the body knows this, which makes healing difficult. However, in Italy, their laws allow them to keep everything intact, including the veins and muscles, which means a more natural bone. Unfortunately, the operation wouldn't be cheap, costing over $100,000, which was money I didn't have. On top of that, I'd need to stay in Italy for several months while I recovered, which meant buying airfares and accommodation, and I'd be away from Tessa, Hunter, and Fawny for that time. Overall, Italy seemed like the best option for healing my leg, but, financially, it was out of reach, so I went ahead with option one – a repeat of my initial surgery. I spent many hours thinking, *Am I crazy to agree to the exact same surgery that just failed?* But I trusted the surgeons and had faith they could save my leg.

I did discuss the possibility of a prosthetic metal shinbone with the surgeons, but they said a prosthetic would only last 1 to 10 years. The problem was, they couldn't just replace it every few years, because they couldn't keep screwing new holes in the bones to hold the prosthetic in place. We needed a more permanent solution. Plus, bone is apparently much stronger than metal. The other problem was, if we put metal in my leg, both the ankle and knee joins would calcify and stop growing altogether, meaning we could never go back to trying a donor bone. Once you go down the list of options, there's no turning back.

Before learning all this, I assumed that super-durable, 3D-printed, prosthetic bones were an option, but the technology doesn't exist, at least not yet. It's often surprising how advanced yet how limited medical science is.

So, once again, I went under the knife, which turned out to be quite traumatic. Since my diagnosis, I'd always had one good leg, and now they were about to cut into it. With that leg, I'd survived, recently managing to live a somewhat normal life – working, playing with Hunter, going to the beach, doing a bit of gym – and now I was putting it all on the line. *When they take the bone, how will it feel? How well will my leg work? Will it work at all? Is it worth the sacrifice?* Regardless of what happened, I'd never have a normal leg again.

Wrapping My Head Around Surgery

Much of my journey has been about sacrifice. I sacrificed footy to help solve my autoimmune issue and continue carpentry. When I was diagnosed with cancer, I sacrificed carpentry. When I agreed to surgery and the wide margins they wanted to cut, I was potentially sacrificing my leg. Now I was being asked to sacrifice another leg, or at least sacrifice its strength, stability, and function.

I spent a lot of time in meetings with my healing team, which consisted of my naturopath Sheryl and my healers Alison and Penny, to prepare myself for what was to come. I never saw any counsellors or psychologists; instead, I took a more holistic approach, relying on my naturopath and healers for guidance. If I was going to do this, I had to go in fully committed. There was no room for hesitation or doubt.

Jake and Mum both offered to donate their fibulas, but it doesn't work that way. It's not like the movies. They don't take bones out of living people to give to someone else. Even if it were allowed, I wouldn't have accepted their offers anyway. The only thing worse than sacrificing my good leg would've been sacrificing someone else's. I love them too much to put them through that.

Surgery Number Three

During the surgery, which took place in August 2022, they cut both legs open from knee to ankle. Once again, I was counting my lucky stars. Not many people can get through two of these surgeries, let alone three. My leg had already experienced so much trauma, and the surgeon said they might need to take skin grafts from other parts of my body if I swelled up too badly. It's so nerve-racking when you're about to get put to sleep and you don't know what you'll be waking up to. It was such a complicated surgery, and so much could go wrong. As they were putting me to sleep, I prayed that I'd get through it, just one more time.

From the bad leg, they removed the donor bone, my repurposed fibula, and all the metalware they'd installed. From the good leg, they took the only fibula left in my body.

This time, instead of placing the fibula alongside the donor bone, they wanted to put it inside, like a hot dog in a bun. Previously, there were big gaps between the donor bone and my own bones at the joins, which was why healing was so difficult. This time, they'd ensure the bone went from top to bottom, leaving as little gap as possible.

So, they added the new bones, redid all the plumbing, installed new metalware, and stitched me up from knee to ankle on both legs. The soft plastic surgeons enjoyed stitching me up because they could match my tattoos together.

When I woke up, the first thing I did was check to make sure I had both legs, which I did, and no cages on, which I didn't. *All right, so far so good.* Once again, I received the post-surgery report, and all was well – a massive relief.

Within two days, they wanted me standing. On the 'good' leg, I'd be able to fully weight-bear, even with the missing fibula. The surgeons promised it wouldn't feel any different. However, I had to be careful with the reconstructed leg until the joins had begun to heal, slowly putting more and more weight on it over time to stimulate bone growth. From what I could tell, the surgery was a success. *Sigh.* I should've known better.

The first time I put weight on my good leg, it felt like I was stepping on broken glass. Pure agony. Suddenly, my good leg wasn't so good anymore. I broke down that day. I felt defeated.

What have I done?

ZACK'S HEALTH AND WELLBEING TIP

USE A HYPERBARIC CHAMBER

As mentioned, hyperbaric oxygen therapy has been an important part of my recovery routine. However, it's not the easiest therapy to access – it's not exactly something you can do at home. You'll either need to get a medical referral (to have some of the cost covered) or pay full price at a private facility.

Either way, the benefits of the hyperbaric chamber are worth pursuing and include increased healing, boosted immune system, and infection reduction.[11] Essentially, it's an all-round health enhancer that has the potential to make a huge impact on recovery.

#9

"

Our greatest weakness lies in giving up. The most certain way to succeed is always to try just one more time.

– THOMAS EDISON

Chapter 10

BUILT UP, KNOCKED DOWN

Walking on Broken Glass

After my third surgery, the pain in my previously good leg refused to go away. It didn't matter that the surgeons had promised it wouldn't feel any different; the reality was that I was in agony whenever I put weight on that leg. I was constantly walking on broken glass.

I'd tried to save one leg, and, in the process, I'd ruined the other.

Did I make the wrong decision? Should I have opted for amputation? Have I sacrificed my one good leg for... I don't even know what yet? I felt so much uncertainty and doubt, and I bawled my eyes out on more than one occasion.

The surgeons told me the pain would eventually fade, but they'd also told me I wouldn't feel it in the first place. I didn't know what to believe anymore. I was scared.

Building Myself Back Up... Again

After three long and difficult months, the pain did fade, and I was able to focus on rehab and building myself back up. I went from a wheelchair to crutches and continued to make progress, putting more and more weight on my reconstructed leg. I was pretty much repeating the same cycle as before, going to the pool each day to do rehab exercises. The pool is the only place where I can take my power back, walking unassisted in waist-deep water and feeling some sense of normality. It's a powerful feeling.

Once I was well enough, I went back to work with Michael, but it didn't last long. Two of his big jobs fell through, and he didn't have any more work for me. So, I finished up with Michael around Christmas of 2022 and began looking for other work.

Michael's former leading hand, Keiran, had left the business to work at an earthmoving company, and he offered me a job driving trucks. The problem was, I didn't have my heavy rigid licence, so I'd need to get it before I could start work.

I called up the training company and explained my situation. "The truck's automatic, and my right leg's fine. I've got a strong upper body, so I can pull myself up into the truck for the test. Can I get my heavy rigid licence?"

"Yeah, sure, I guess... There are no rules stopping you. If you can get in a truck fine, I can't see why not."

I threw myself in the deep end, learning to drive a truck and earning my heavy rigid licence. Once again, I was focused on what I could do, not what I couldn't.

I felt anxious about starting a new job. New crew, new faces – what would they think of a guy on crutches showing up to a job site? But the crutches don't symbolise who I am. Once I'm in a truck or an excavator, I'm as useful as the next guy – and I'd prove it. Once the guys heard my story and understood what I'd been through, they saw past the crutches and welcomed me onto the crew. I had no reason to be anxious at all.

Over time, I got up to 80 percent weight bearing on the reconstructed leg, which was the most progress I'd ever made. It was the most it had ever healed, and I only needed one crutch to get around. Finally, I was starting to regain some semblance of a normal life.

Then I got assaulted.

Just a Normal Night at the Pub… or So I Thought

One group of mates and I had formed a punter's club, and we'd try to get together as much as possible, which is hard when everyone has work and family commitments. One night, however, we managed to line up a bit of a get-together at a local pub for our annual punter's meeting. The plan was dinner and drinks.

Jake, my best mate Luke, and I met four other guys from the group at around 4 pm. The boys put a few bets on, and we had dinner and a couple drinks. Due to my health issues, I didn't drink for over two years, and even now I rarely do. Eventually, the other boys left due to other commitments, and Jake, Luke, and I stayed.

Luke's AFL team, Adelaide, was playing that night, so we moved closer to the TV in the main bar area to watch the game.

At some point, a group of rough-looking guys walked in. They were being loud, carrying on like idiots, but we minded our own business and kept our heads down. We weren't looking for any trouble. The guys looked like they'd come from the local footy and already had a few drinks under their belts when they showed up at the pub. We didn't think too much of it and continued to chat and watch the game.

Eventually, at around 10 pm, the game ended, and the part of the pub where we were sitting was closing up. There was, however, still a raised deck area that was still open. As we were moving from one spot to another, I ran into a chippie I'd met through work, so I sat at the pool tables chatting with him. While I chatted, Jake and Luke moved to the deck area about 15 metres away. The deck was about eight stairs high, basically head height.

"What's the story with your leg?" the chippie asked, and I started explaining everything.

According to Luke, one of the guys from the rough-looking group approached Jake and started taunting him. "Oh, we've got a tough bloke over here."

Jake was confused, as he hadn't done anything to provoke the guy. "What do you mean?"

"You think you're tough, do ya?"

"What are you talking about? We're just here for a couple of drinks, minding our own business. We don't want any trouble," Jake said, putting his hands up to show he didn't want to fight. But the guy kept harassing him, going on and on, hoping to get a reaction. "Mate, I'm here with my brother. We're here for a good time. No one needs to get hurt. Just leave it." But the guy kept going.

Luke approached one of the other guys from the group and asked him to come and sort his mate out. The second guy came over and put a hand on his mate's chest. "Leave these boys alone, they're all right." He was a big bloke and could've done more to stop his mate. As we were about to find out, a hand on the chest just didn't cut it.

The first guy moved around his mate's hand and hit Jake with a headbutt. By this time, the rest of the group had arrived and was surrounding Jake, who realised they were about to go to town on him, so, in an act of self-preservation, he hit the guy back.

Fight or Flight

I, oblivious to what was happening, heard a loud bang. *What was that?* Looking around for the source of the sound, I saw Jake lying on the floor of the deck. Someone had hit him hard enough to knock him down. He didn't look well. *Oh, no.* It was instant shock. After everything I've been through, I don't have any anger or violence inside me. I prefer to just walk away. That night, I had a choice to make: I could either sit back and do nothing, or I could put my leg at risk to help my brother.

I threw my crutch aside and hobbled across the pub to the deck, labouring up the stairs. When I got there, the first guy was standing over Jake, shouting, "Get up, you cunt. Get up!" – so I hit him. I didn't do it to hurt the guy; I just wanted the pressure off Jake so he could get up and get away. In response, about four of them started hitting me, knocking me to the floor. Once I was on the floor, they kept going, hitting and kicking me while I was down. All I could do was lie there, cover up as much as possible, and try not to get knocked out. I was waiting for a stomp to the face, thinking I'd wake up in the hospital. At that point, everything went silent, foggy. I couldn't hear a thing. Then, suddenly, I could hear *everything*.

"Get off him!" Girls were screaming. Tables and chairs were crashing around us. Other people were shouting. It was chaos. I couldn't get up, so I kept waiting and waiting for help to come, but none came. If I tried to get up, it would leave my face open and vulnerable to copping more damage. The pub's security didn't want to get involved. We were on our own.

Eventually, some locals jumped in and tried to pull the guys off us, but they ended up getting assaulted too. With tables being flipped and chairs being thrown, the scene was surreal. It was like an over-the-top bar fight in a movie. I've since seen footage of the incident, and I couldn't even see myself at that point. They were all over me.

The Chaos Continues

While the pressure was off Jake, he managed to crawl off to the side and escape the worst of the onslaught, for a moment at least. However, when he saw them beating the crap out of me, he crawled on top of me to shield me from the blows, taking hit after hit after hit to the back of the head.

Suddenly, I felt myself being dragged, and I looked up to see what was happening. It was Luke, pulling me from the brawl. I looked back at Jake. He was still on the floor, with some guy kicking him in the face.

"You've got to help Jake," I said, blood dripping from my busted face.

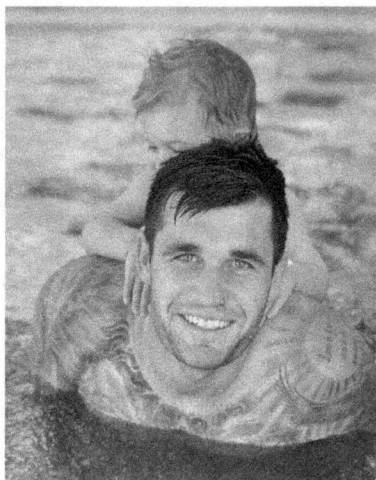

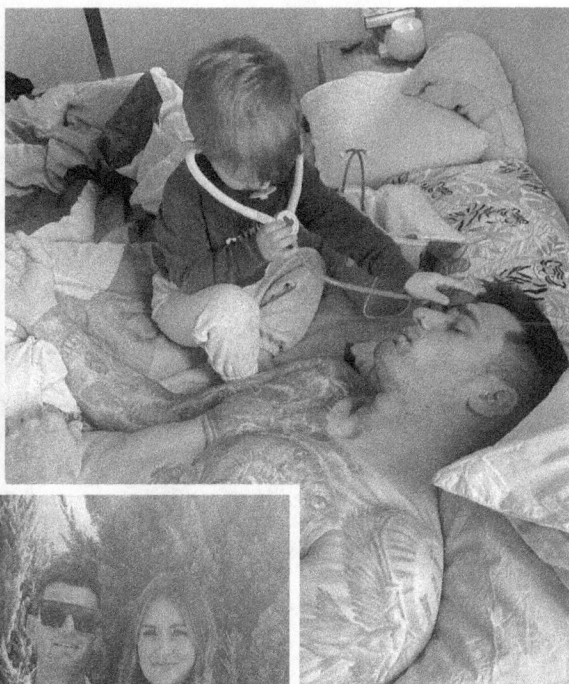

Recovery, family,
and a check-up
from Dr Hunter.

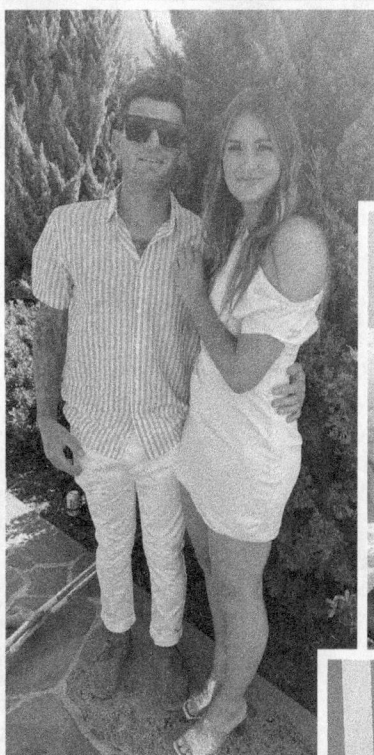

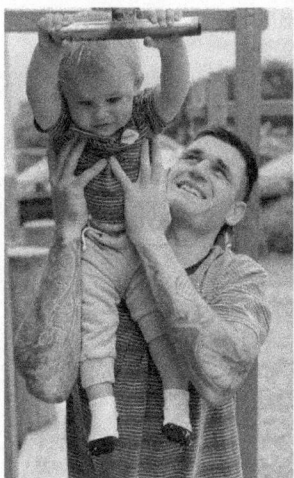

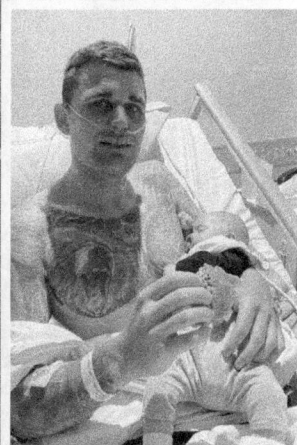

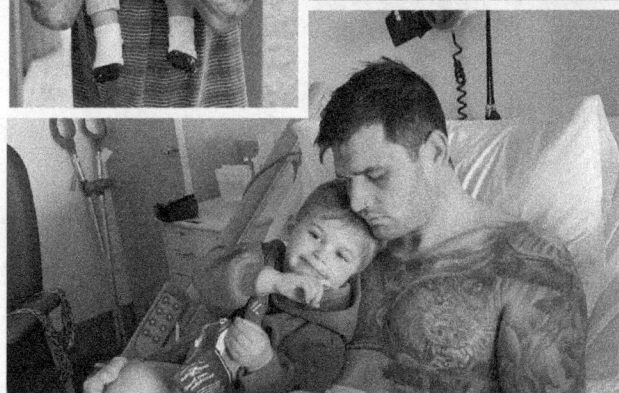

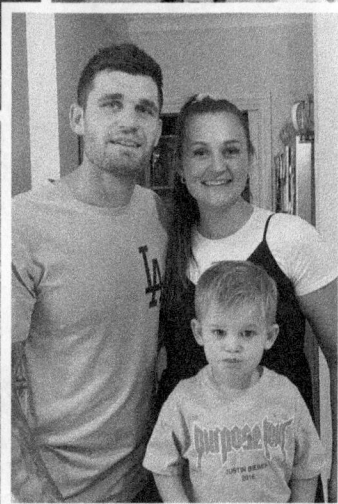

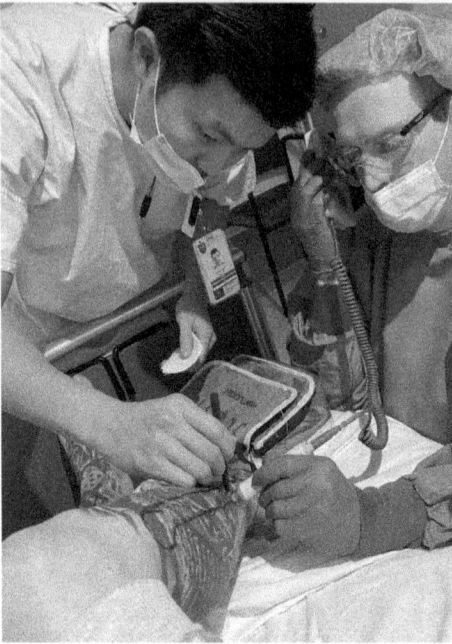

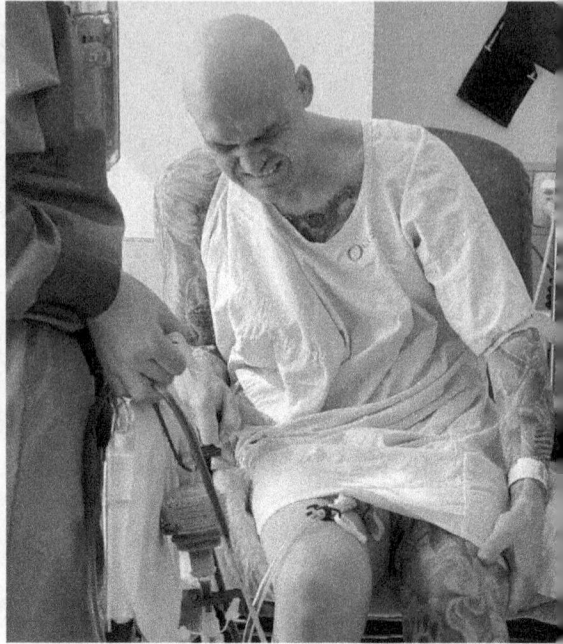

First surgery to remove Zack's 'lump'.

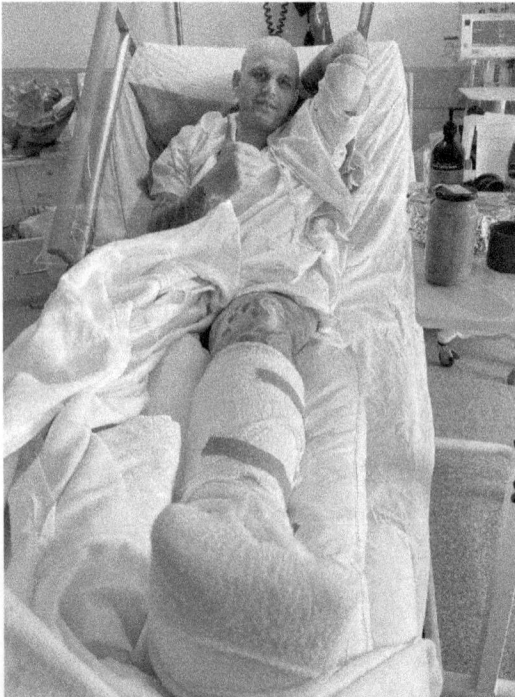

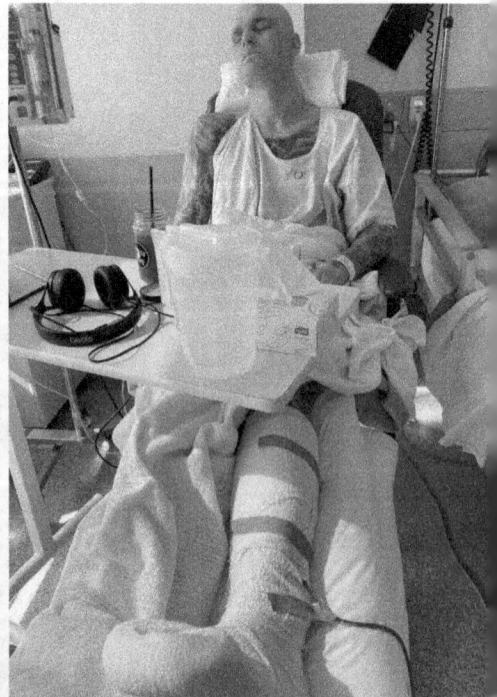

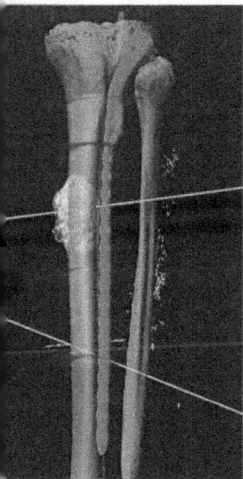

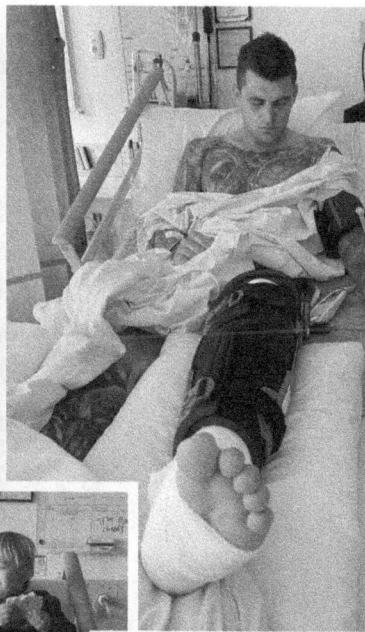

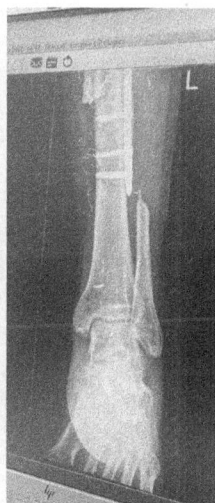

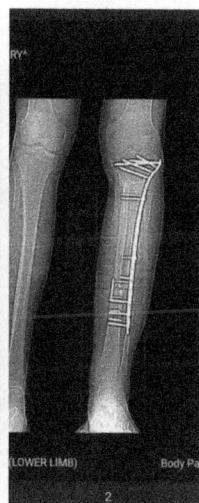

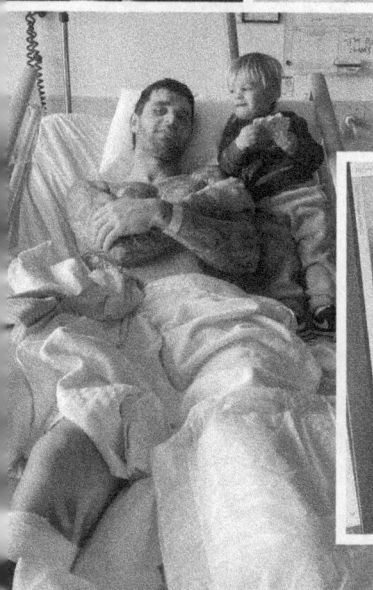

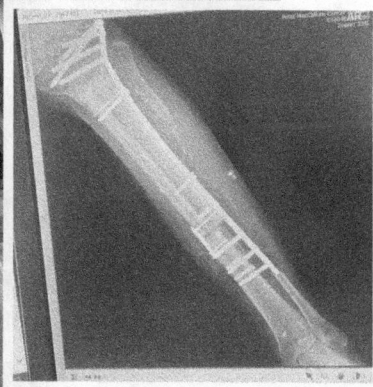

X-rays, operations,
and more hospital time.

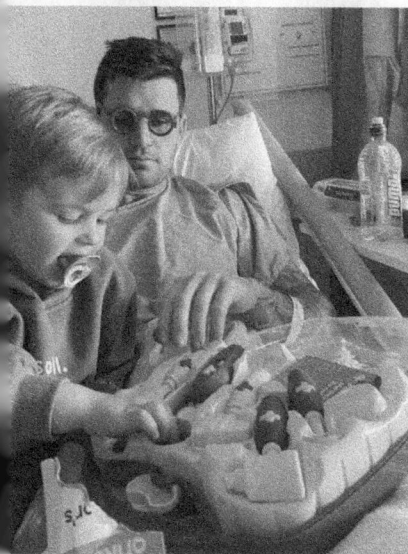

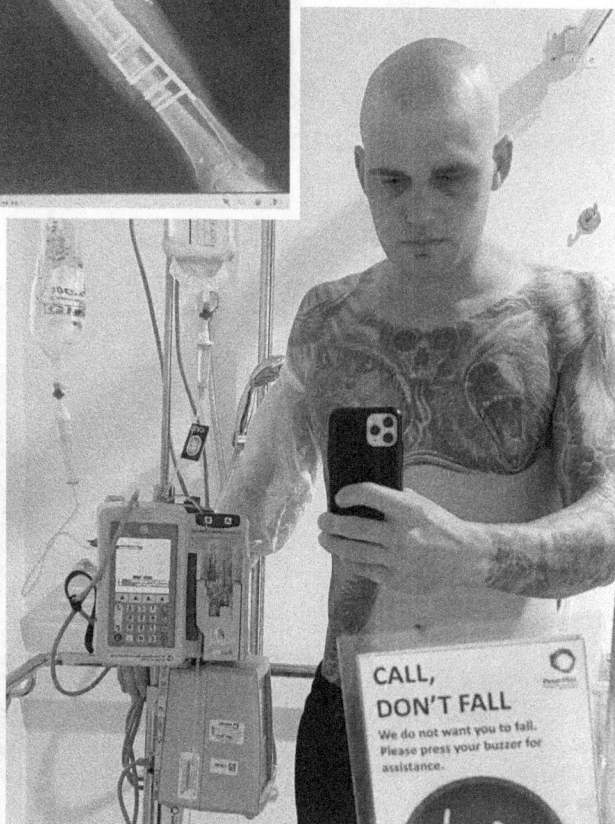

CALL,
DON'T FALL
We do not want you to fall.
Please press your buzzer for
assistance.

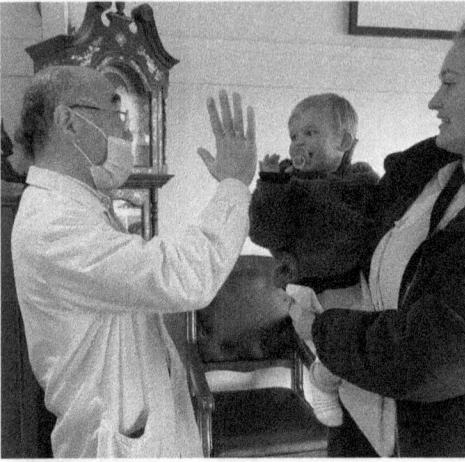

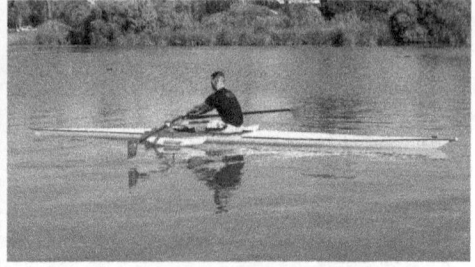

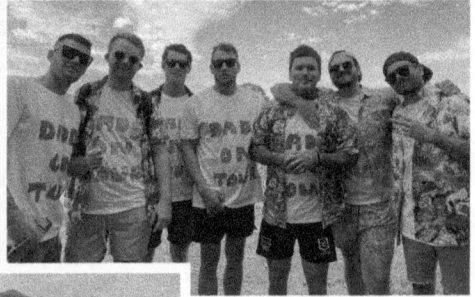

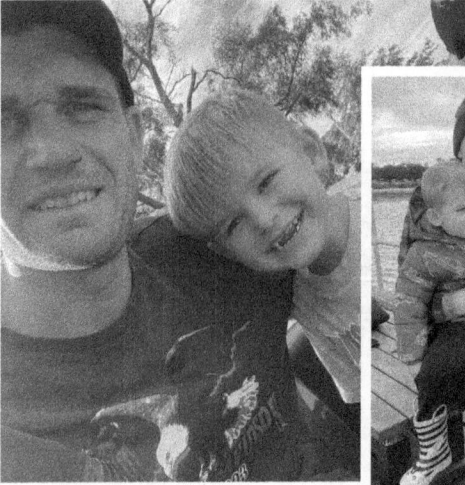

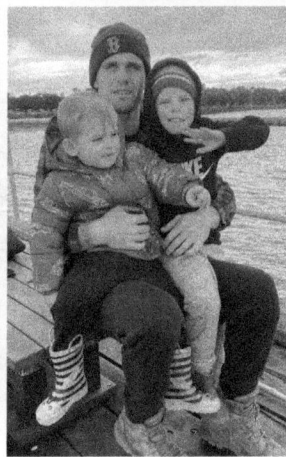

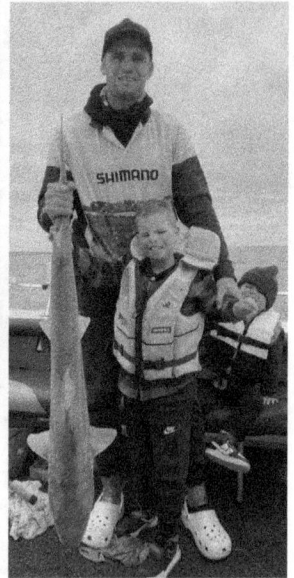

Cancer-free and living life to its fullest.

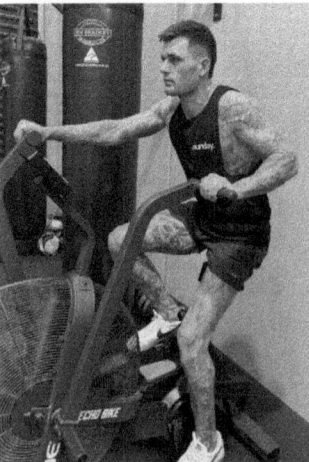

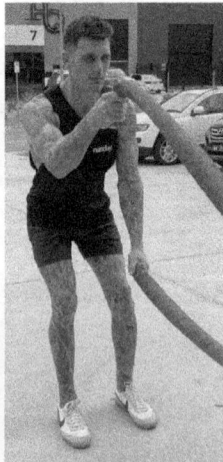

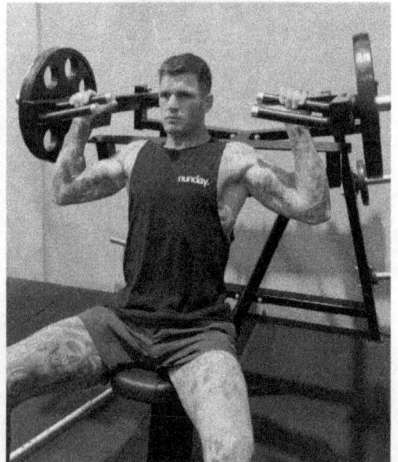

Luke and I went back into the brawl, and I grabbed the guy's leg to stop him from kicking Jake, which gave one of the locals enough time to drag him away. In the chaos, I managed to get away too.

As Luke helped Jake get farther away, I lost sight of them. I was hobbling around the pub, dazed and confused. I didn't know where my crutch was, so I was forced to keep putting weight on my reconstructed leg. As I searched the pub, the fight continued. It had moved off the deck area, and the group that had assaulted me and Jake was now fighting its way through the pub. *What is even happening?*

I hobbled over to a security guard who was sitting by the door ignoring it all. "Are you going to get in there?" The look on his face said 'no'.

Eventually, the brawl calmed down, but the guy who'd started the fight was like a rabid dog – he wanted to keep going – and his mate had to grab him in a bear hug and drag him out. He was frothing at the mouth, wanting to inflict more pain.

As I hobbled around, still looking for Jake and Luke, a girl came over and handed me my crutch. "Are you okay?" she asked.

"Where's my brother?"

"He's out the front, he's safe. You've got to get out of here."

I made my way outside, but Jake wasn't there. I did, however, meet the chippie I'd been talking to when the fight started. As it turned out, it was him and his mates who were trying to pull the guys off us. For his efforts, he received a busted-up face and a broken nose – it was practically sideways.

"Thanks so much for trying to save us," I said.

"I'd do it again," he said. "It's so wrong that they'd fight someone for no reason and beat up a guy on crutches. I don't stand for that at all."

We moved away from the pub, looking for Jake, eventually finding him down the road, standing on the corner of the street. "We've got to get out of here," I said. His face was all beaten up, and he had welts all over his head – he was a complete mess. I probably didn't look much better.

The chippie's girlfriend got us in her car and drove us to a nearby McDonald's so we could take a moment to breathe, have a drink, gather our thoughts, and try to figure out what the hell had happened. Somehow, we'd gone from having a good night out to having the shit kicked out of us. At that point, I knew I'd copped a beating, but I didn't know exactly what the damage was.

Note: The incident at the pub is currently under police investigation.

Assessing the Damage

Jake and I got a lift home and went straight into the bathroom, trying to wash the blood off us. After assessing the damage, it was clear that I had a broken nose and Jake had taken some heavy hits to the head.

Tessa, who'd been in bed, heard the noise and came to investigate. She turned on the lights and looked us over, shocked, confused. "What the hell happened?"

I explained what had gone down at the pub and that I had a broken nose. At this stage, I didn't know if my leg had taken any damage.

Although I needed to get my leg checked and get facial scans, I couldn't go to the hospital right away. The assault happened on a Saturday night, and I did disability support every Sunday, helping Taj, a disabled boy, often taking him camping and fishing and doing other outdoor activities. He never knew his dad, so I've tried to fill that role as much as I can. It's all part of giving back after receiving so much help when I was at my lowest points.

After getting sick and undergoing countless surgeries, I needed support daily from friends and family. Before that, I was always the helper or provider to my loved ones, but suddenly it was their turn to look after me. It was very hard to let go of that role and accept help from others. I suffered a lot of guilt around people having to do so much for me for so long, and I still work on myself daily to deal with those negative emotions.

Once I was on track to recovery and in a more stable state of mind, I realised I wanted to give back to not just my family and friends but also to others who needed help. When I met Taj, I decided I wanted to be more than his support worker. I wanted to be a male role model, someone he could look up to. I wanted to guide him on his disability journey and show him he can defy the odds and get through any challenges thrown his way.

Taj has taught me that materialistic things don't matter. Just being present, enjoying what we have, and appreciating the small things in life is all it takes to be happy. Taj is hearing-impaired, but that doesn't stop him from communicating with others and being enthusiastic about learning important life skills. Each day we spend together, I'm amazed at his resilience and persistence. He has helped Hunter learn to be kind to everyone and not judge people blindly. Hunter just sees Taj as a friend; he doesn't see his disability. Hunter has also learnt little pieces of sign language, which is a powerful life skill to have. If I can make a difference in Taj's life, it will help me heal my own trauma and give me a new purpose – helping others. I can relate to Taj. He's a fighter who defied the odds when the doctors counted him out. I'm truly grateful he came into my life. After leaving carpentry behind, I didn't think I'd find purpose again, but now I've found my true calling, and I can't thank Taj enough.

The day after the assault was a Sunday, and Taj's mum, Tammie, was relying on me to be there to spend time with her son, so, in the morning, I had to show up at their house with a busted face and a broken nose. I'm not the type of guy who gets in fights, so it was a bit embarrassing. I wanted to be a role model for Tammie's boys, not rock up to their house like I did. I just didn't want to let them down. Currently, I still see Taj three times a week, and I intend to stay in his life for as long as he needs me.

Later that day, I went to the hospital to check the damage. I had no idea how many times I'd been hit, or even where I'd been hit. To check for any internal damage, I had scans done on my head, as did Jake. Aside from the broken nose, I was all clear. Then I explained my situation and asked if they could also check my leg. *Please let nothing be wrong.*

No major breaks, just two broken screws. *Shit.* Those screws were supposed to be holding my leg together. After coming so far, suddenly I was at serious risk of losing my leg. I panicked and discharged myself from Frankston Hospital. In an instant, years of hard work had been ruined by a bunch of drunken idiots.

ZACK'S HEALTH AND WELLBEING TIP

CONNECT TO THE EARTH VIA GROUNDING

You might be asking, *What's grounding?* Put simply, grounding (aka earthing) is the practice of physically touching the earth, therefore, connecting to its natural electrical charge.

Next, you might be asking, *What are the benefits of grounding?* Great question! Research shows that grounding can improve overall health and wellbeing by reducing pain and inflammation, boosting the immune system, and improving the body's ability to heal.[12]

Finally, at this point, it would be fair to ask, *How exactly do I ground myself?* That's the beauty of grounding – it's one of the simplest things you can do to improve your health. All you need to do is make skin contact with the natural earth, for example, by walking barefoot on the grass or along the beach. It's as simple as that.

I practise grounding every day, and it has been a big part of my healing journey. It's simple, effective, and feels great.

#10

"

Do not judge me
by my successes,
judge me by how
many times I fell
down and got
back up again.

– NELSON MANDELA

Chapter 11

DOWN BUT NOT OUT

It's Normal, They Said

To properly assess the damage to my reconstructed leg, I was admitted to St Vincent's Hospital, where they did several scans and concluded that everything was fine.

"My leg's moving," I said. "It's not meant to move like that."

"Oh, a bit of movement is normal. If there are any issues, come back in a month or two and we'll do some more scans."

"Something's not right," I said. But the doctors reassured me that my leg was holding together and sent me home.

A week later, I went to Peter Mac and demanded to see my surgeon. My gut told me that something wasn't right.

All for Nothing

"How does this feel?" Claudia asked, pushing on my leg.

"Look how this is moving," I said, pointing to a part of my shin that absolutely *shouldn't* have been moving.

"Yeah, I thought that might be the case. This needs to be reconstructed."

It was like being smacked in the head again. After trying to protect my brother, trying to do the right thing, everything I'd worked for had been taken away from me. I'd

DOWN BUT NOT OUT

already sacrificed my remaining fibula for the last surgery. I didn't have another to spare. How would another reconstruction even be possible? *I'm going to lose my leg,* I thought. *After everything I've done, I'm going to lose my leg.*

"Can you fix it and save my leg? What if you replace the two broken screws?"

"It's… more technical than that."

Unfortunately, they couldn't just go in and do some quick maintenance. If they tightened the metal plate in my leg, which they needed to do, it would kink certain veins and cut off circulation to my leg. Whatever they decided to do, the solution wouldn't be simple. Each day, I thought, *Please be able to fix it. Please don't cut off my leg. This can't be it. This can't be the end. Please save my leg.*

The constant setbacks took a toll on my mental health. There I was, at one point, doing earthmoving, going to the gym regularly, building myself back up – 40, 60, 80 percent – only to get knocked back ten spaces. Finally, I'd felt like I had a normal life at my fingertips, and it was wrenched away, just like that. All the normality I had regained was gone in an instant.

Mentally, it was very tough to deal with, and it was something I had to work through to ensure I was ready to have another crack at healing my leg.

The Best of the Best on My Case

The best surgeons in the country were working on my case. For several weeks, they had regular meetings, trying to come up with a solution. The goal was to fix my leg without cutting off the blood supply. Without a spare fibula, a full reconstruction wasn't an option. I needed a miracle fix.

Every two weeks, Claudia would call me to explain that they hadn't found a solution. The more time that passed, the more certain I was that I'd lose my leg. *This leg's gone,* I thought. Suddenly, I was faced with the unknown again, but I tried to keep a level head. I kept up with my health and wellness practices while hoping for a miracle. It was all I could do.

Finally, on the sixth week, I saw Sarah, a trauma surgeon at St Vincent's Hospital, who had a possible solution. "We need to put a plate on the inner side of your leg and hope that when we open you up, the vein isn't in the way. If it is, we go to plan B, which would involve putting bolts through your leg, along with a cage around it to clamp everything together. While we're in there, we might as well put some more bone between the joins. This time, we'll take it from your hip."

New surgeon, new ideas. I was hopeful, but also concerned. There was no guarantee any of this would work. On top of that, a hip graft is extremely painful. But, at that point, I'd been in near-constant agony for years – what was a little more if it meant saving my leg? Still, I wasn't exactly enthusiastic about the operation.

Surgery Number Four... When Will It End?

Once again, I was under the knife, being cut from knee to ankle. They took all the metalwear out that was holding my leg together, replaced it with a new plate, and put a second plate on the inside of my leg to support the bottom join, which broke during the assault. Oh, and they also cut a chunk of bone from my hip.

When I woke up, I didn't have a cage around my leg. *That has to be a good sign.* As it turned out, once they opened me up, they found that they could *just* fit a small plate where it needed to go, so no bolts, no cage. They had also successfully placed the 'bonecrete' made from my hip graft between the two joins. However, they couldn't get the two broken screws out of my ankle, as they would have needed to core them out, taking too much bone. "Your leg has gone through enough trauma," one of the surgeons said. "Let's just leave the screws in and give your leg the best chance to heal. We'll worry about them later down the track." It seemed like the operation was a success, but there was one problem – I couldn't feel my legs. *Am I paralysed?*

Luckily, I *wasn't* paralysed; I was under the effects of an epidural, which they'd given me for the pain in my hip. Apparently, it wouldn't be pleasant when the drug wore off, but, for now, I couldn't feel a thing.

So, was the surgery a *complete* success? Not quite.

Due to all the scar tissue from multiple surgeries, visibility wasn't great, and the surgeon accidentally cut a vein, so they had to replace it with a vein from my forearm. Hey, it couldn't *all* go smoothly.

Overall, the operation was a success. *Thank God.* Now, I could get back to healing.

Surgery Aftermath

Three days after surgery, the epidural fully wore off, and I could feel my legs again. Unfortunately, I could also feel the pain in my hip – and it was excruciating. Now I understood why they'd given me the epidural. The pain from the graft was some of the worst I'd ever felt – like I'd been hit by a car. Taking that small chunk of bone from my hip was almost as painful as having my shinbone removed. I couldn't believe it. Not only was my leg sore after the surgery, but the pain in my hip was bordering on unbearable. It was a double dose of agony. I lay flat on my back, not wanting to move a centimetre, as it would set off the pain in my hip.

I ended up spending a week and a half in hospital. Before I could be discharged, I had to prove I could safely use crutches to get around. I was still in a lot of pain, and nothing felt easy, but I had to get home to my son. That was always at the forefront of my mind. *I'll do whatever it takes to get home to Hunter.*

My Reason to Fight

After each major surgery and every major setback, Hunter saw his dad pick himself up and fight another day. I believe that resilience is one of the most powerful tools you can give to a child, or anyone.

Becoming a father gave me a love I didn't know existed. It gave me purpose, a reason to do my best each day, and fuel to fight for my leg. Being a dad has taught me a lot about myself. Hunter brings out the best in me. I've been so broken I wanted to give up and make my pain and suffering go away but as soon as I look into Hunter's beautiful eyes and hear him call me 'Dad', all my issues disappear.

Before his birth and after we learnt that Tessa was pregnant, I prayed each day to make it through so I could live to see his first breath and hold him in my arms. Now, every day is a bonus, and I'm so grateful to be able to watch him grow and achieve his dreams.

I want to be my son's hero. I'm trying to lead by example with my actions, with my dedication to my health, and with rehab to save my leg. When Hunter faces adversity, which he certainly will in life, he knows to never give up – because I never did.

Nothing Can Beat Me

Eventually, I'd made enough progress to be discharged from the hospital, and I was finally back at home with my family, where I could return to my routine, good diet, and healing protocols. I was itching to get back in the ice bath, which always made me feel better mentally and reduced inflammation. Once again, recovery became my primary focus.

I had beaten autoimmunity. I had beaten cancer. I would beat a broken leg. I had come too far to accept failure as an option. For myself, for my family, for everyone who supported me on my healing journey, I *would* walk again. I was determined to create a happy ending for my story, and, after all I'd been through, nothing could stand in my way.

I was unbeatable.

ZACK'S HEALTH AND WELLBEING TIP

EXERCISE REGULARLY

Being on crutches, I found it difficult to exercise. When I was experiencing the worst of the chemo side effects, I found it impossible. However, as soon as I was able, I was back in the gym, doing what I could to rebuild my body and mind.

Exercise is great for not only physical health but mental health as well.[13] If you want to feel at your best mentally, physical exercise is a must. Personally, going to the gym has been massively positive for my mental health. I go 3 to 5 times a week, even if it's only to do 20 minutes on the bike, the rowing machine, or to do rehab exercises. I also do pool rehab 2 to 3 times a week. Essentially, rehabilitation and getting back in shape has become a full-time job.

If you're someone who could benefit from a personal trainer, I say go for it. I train with a guy named Giani several times a week, and he has given me the confidence to not put barriers up just because I'm on crutches. I can still go into the gym and do the work – no excuses!

#11

"

The best way to not feel hopeless is to get up and do something. Don't wait for good things to happen to you. If you go out and make some good things happen, you will fill the world with hope, you will fill yourself with hope.

– BARACK OBAMA

THE PATH I NOW WALK

Life Prepares Us for Every Challenge

Looking back, while trying to solve my autoimmune issue, everything I learnt about health and wellness, all the alternative therapies, lifestyle changes, and dietary habits were preparing me for what was to come. If I was going to beat cancer, I needed to throw everything I had at it, and, by then, I had a pretty decent toolkit. My diet was clean; I'd removed many toxins from my environment; I understood the power of fasting, and I took Chinese herbs daily, along with my naturopathic supplements, never missing a beat.

The thing is, I didn't just wake up and start doing these things one day. I didn't instantly understand how to live a healthy lifestyle. All of these changes took place over several years. It was a long but totally worthwhile learning process. Ultimately, when the cancer struck, I was ready to fight. If I hadn't had such a tough battle with the autoimmunity, I might not have been so well-prepared.

But I didn't beat cancer alone – far from it. Everything, big and small, that everyone did and continues to do to support me on my healing journey got me where I am today. They kept my head above water when I barely had the strength to stay afloat myself. I have a deep love and appreciation for all the people in my life. Without a doubt, having them in my life saved my life.

Why I Share My Story

Why did I write this book? Because I've been to hell and back several times over and lived to write about it. I could've given up at any moment, but I didn't, and now my life is more beautiful and meaningful than ever. My leg is still healing, and, while nothing is certain yet, I've made good progress. Even so, I'm not sitting around waiting for it to heal before I continue living. I'm out there living my life now, filling it with purpose, hoping to inspire others to keep fighting, no matter what. This book isn't just my story; it's a source of hope for anyone who's going through hard times. I want to change lives, save lives, just like the people around me saved mine. I want to give back as much as possible. It's the least I could do. When searching for solutions, I want people to leave no stone unturned, fighting till the end and doing everything in their power to stay healthy. I want people to know that if they focus on prevention, there'll be no need for a cure.

So, What Now?

While I have my health and my beautiful family, I need something more to fill my core. I need lofty goals. I need a greater purpose. I needed a new challenge.

After sacrificing so much, I missed playing sport. I loved competing and being part of a team, and I wanted that in my life again. While I know I'll never play footy again, that doesn't mean I can't do something. Why focus on what I can't do? There's plenty I *can* do. Footy, no, but something... *Maybe I could qualify for the Paralympics.* Hey, why not dream big? Whether my leg heals or I end up with a prosthetic, that's my goal – to compete in the Paralympics. I've already started training. Right now, the plan is to apply for rowing because it doesn't require the use of legs. In fact, I just qualified for seated para-athletic events, which is very exciting.

I've beaten cancer; now it's time to see what else I'm capable of. I'm not just doing it for me, either. I feel like I owe it to my family and everyone else who supported me to make the most of my life, the one I almost lost.

I'm also keeping up with my alternative therapies, although I space my naturopathy and Qigong healing sessions out a lot more now. I also get checked monthly to ensure I'm still in good health. I still keep a clean diet, and I'm in the ice bath every day, maintaining the mental toughness I've built over the years. I also do visualisation exercises every day in the ice bath, visualising taking Fawn for a walk for the first time in years, being Hunter's soccer coach, and walking Tessa down the aisle. They're things I want to happen in the future, but I'm visualising them as if they're happening now so my body gets the message – *We must heal this leg.*

On top of my Paralympic dream, I plan to keep sharing my story, speaking from stages and inspiring others to find that inner strength they might not know they have. On my journey, I've learnt exactly how unbeatable we can be when we're willing to fight, and I want to share this knowledge with anyone who needs it. Let my struggle be your strength.

After everything I've been through, I'm not just sitting around feeling sorry for myself. I'm always setting goals. I'm always moving forward.

You Are Unbeatable

Much of my journey involved letting go and trusting the process. While I did take additional alternative measures to support my health, I had to trust the medical professionals that were there to support me. Of course, I did eventually draw the line, but not until I was absolutely sure it was the right thing to do.

The entire time, I was wrestling with the unknown. As humans, we often fear the unknown. We prefer life to be predictable, comfortable, safe. However, when we push through the difficult and uncomfortable moments, we build resilience, and I've built a truckload over the years. What could possibly faze me now? I'm unbeatable. And guess what? You are too.

The hard truth is, you can have the best support team possible, but you're the only one who can truly pick yourself up when you're down. We all need support in difficult times. However, at the end of the day, it's your own resilience, grit, and determination that will get you through. You must be prepared to fight and never accept defeat.

The tough times have the ability to either make us or break us. Don't let them break you. I'm living proof that it's always worth fighting, even when the odds are stacked heavily against us. That's when we truly get to show who we are and what we're made of. I've been broken many times, but the sun always rises the next day, so get back up and keep fighting the fight.

If you're going through tough times, fighting to survive, don't stop. Surviving, getting to the other side is well worth the effort. I know it because I've lived it, and I hope my story lets you know it too. My best advice is to keep someone close to your heart to drive you to never give up and give you the fuel to keep fighting. Because it's *always* worth fighting.

Want to join me on my journey? Let's connect on social media. Follow me on Instagram (@zacks.journey) or get in touch through my website zacksjourney.org.

A Time to Reflect

Sometimes, after reading a book, I like to reflect with some questions to really cement the ideas in my head. If you're also a fan of reflection, here are some questions to get you started.

1. What's one thing you can take from this book and implement in your daily life?

_____

_____

_____

2. When you're having a bad day or going through a tough time, who is someone you can reach out to for support?

_____

_____

_____

3. What part of this book had the biggest impact on you or inspired you the most?

_____

_____

_____

4. What goals will you set to improve your life after reading this book?

_____

_____

_____

5. Which of my health protocols did you find the most interesting and plan to add to your routine?

_____

_____

_____

6. What's a strategy discussed in this book that you can use when facing life's biggest challenges?

_____

_____

_____

7. Do you have a friend or family member who could benefit from this book? If so, let them know!

_____

_____

_____

Acknowledgements

I'd like to thank my local community, family, and friends who supported me on my journey and donated towards my GoFundMe campaign so I could continue buying my Chinese medicine to keep healthy and beat cancer. I'll be forever grateful for your generosity and having you guys in my life.

I also want to give a shout-out to the people I listen to on podcasts to get vital health tips and inspiration to be a better person each day and keep me on track. Ed Mylett, Jay Shetty, Tony Robbins, Joe Dispenza, Gary Brecka, and Don Tolman – thank you!

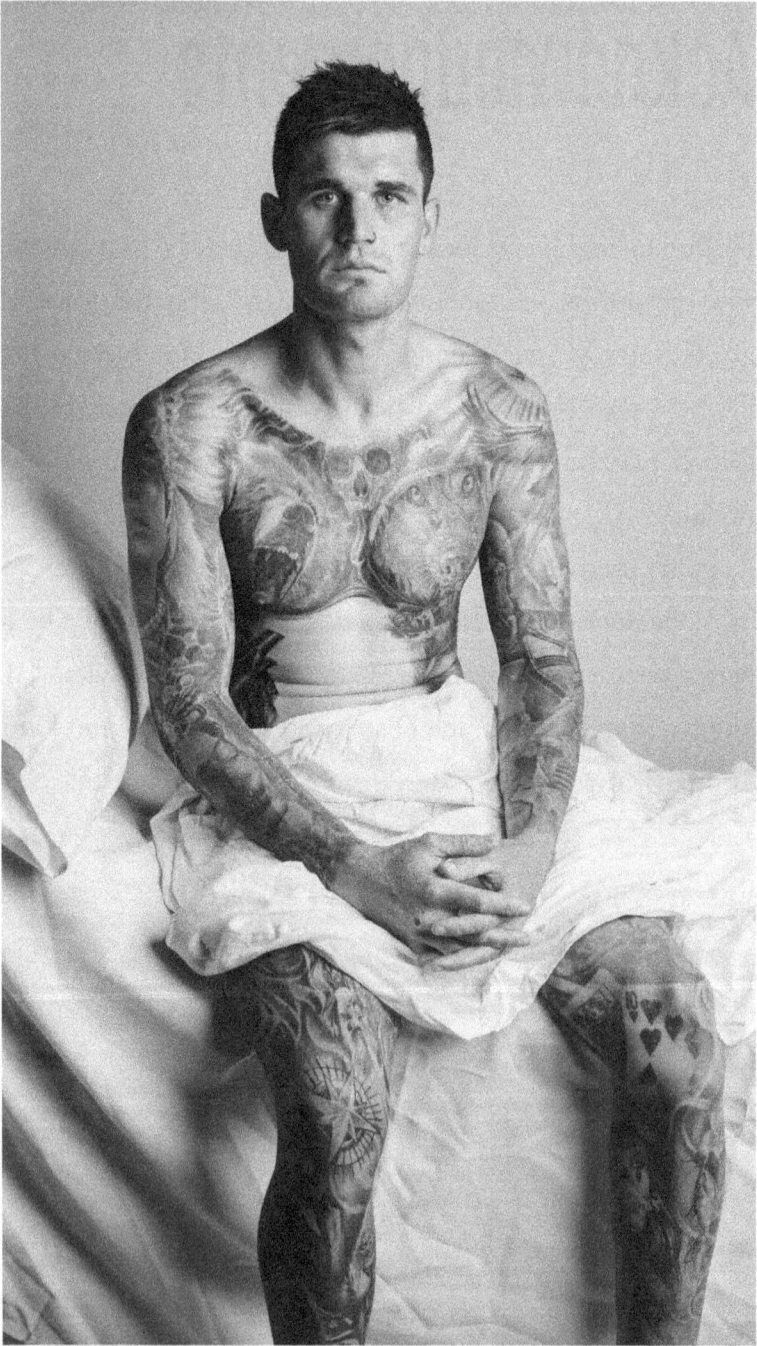

About the Author

Zack Condick is an author, athlete, professional speaker, and cancer survivor.

When an autoimmune issue cut short a promising career in Aussie rules football, Zack channelled his passion into his carpentry business. However, after being diagnosed with a rare bone cancer with low odds of survival, he was forced to give up his business to fight for his life.

Determined to defy the odds, Zack explored alternative therapies to complement his conventional treatment of gruelling chemotherapy and complicated surgeries. The complex and relentless nature of his condition meant he was at real risk of losing his leg, and he had to fight every step of the way to keep it. With the birth of his son Hunter, Zack found a new purpose, a new reason to keep fighting.

Now Zack's mission is to give back in every way possible. Discovering a passion for disability support, he helps others through their own challenges, providing support and a strong role model to those who need it. By sharing his story, Zack aims to inspire others experiencing adversity and extreme hardship to keep fighting, no matter the odds. He knows the fight isn't over until you say it is.

Although limited by his leg, Zack still has a passion for sport, and he is training to one day compete in the Paralympics.

He enjoys fishing, camping, and spending time in the outdoors. To Zack, family is everything, and his son Hunter, partner Tessa, and dog Fawn are the lights of his life. After everything he has been through, he cherishes every moment he gets to spend with them.

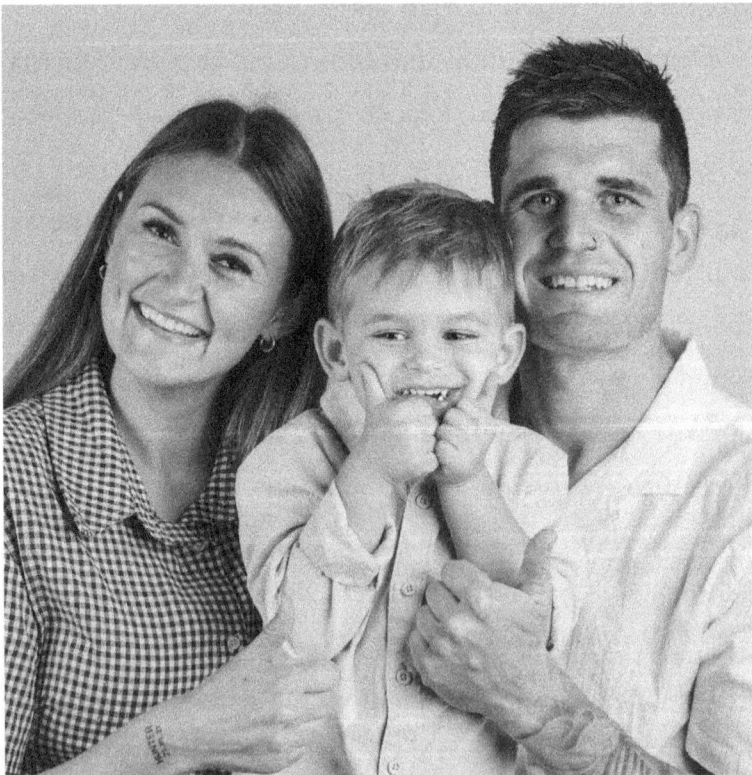

Endnotes

1   Peng, Y, Ao, M, Dong, B, Jiang, Y, Yu, L, Chen, Z, Hu, C, & Xu, R 2021, 'Anti-Inflammatory Effects of Curcumin in the Inflammatory Diseases: Status, Limitations and Countermeasures', *Drug Design, Development and Therapy*, vol 15, pp 4503-4525, viewed 23 February 2024, doi.org/10.2147/DDDT. S327378.

2   Horne, BD, Muhlestein, JB, Lappé, DL, May, HT, Carlquist, JF, Galenko, O, Brunisholz, KD, & Anderson, JL 2013, 'Randomized Cross-Over Trial of Short-Term Water-Only Fasting: Metabolic and Cardiovascular Consequences', *Nutrition, Metabolism, and Cardiovascular Diseases,* vol 23, no 11, pp 1050-1057, doi.org/10.1016/j.numecd.2012.09.007.

3   De Cabo, R & Mattson, MP 2019, 'Effects of Intermittent Fasting on Health, Aging, and Disease', *New England Journal of Medicine,* vol 381, no 26, pp 2541-2551, viewed 23 February 2024, doi.org/10.1056/NEJMra1905136.

4   HUMIRA n.d., 'Important Safety Information', *AbbVie,* viewed 10 February 2023, https://www.humira.com/crohns/safety-side-effects.

5   Kandel, S 2019, 'An Evidence-Based Look at the Effects of Diet on Health', *Cureus,* vol 11, no 5, viewed 23 February 2024, doi.org/10.7759/cureus.4715.

6   Simonsmeier, BA, Androniea, M, Buecker, S, & Frank, C 2020. 'The Effects of Imagery Interventions in Sports: A Meta-Analysis', *International Review of Sport and Exercise Psychology*, viewed 23 February 2024, doi.org/10.1080/17509 84X.2020.1780627.

7   Myers, SP & Vigar, V 2019, 'The State of the Evidence for Whole-System, Multi-Modality Naturopathic Medicine: A Systematic Scoping Review', *Journal of Alternative and Complementary Medicine,* vol 25, no 2, pp 141-168, viewed 23 February 2024, doi.org/10.1089/acm.2018.0340.

8   Xiang, Y, Guo, Z, Zhu, P, Chen, J, & Huang, Y 2019, 'Traditional Chinese Medicine as a Cancer Treatment: Modern Perspectives of Ancient but Advanced

Science', *Cancer Medicine*, vol 8, no 5, pp 1958-1975, viewed 23 February 2024, doi.org/10.1002/cam4.2108.

9   Sharma, H 2015, 'Meditation: Process and Effects', *Ayu*, vol 36, no 3, pp 233-237, viewed 25 February 2024, doi.org/10.4103/0974-8520.182756.

10   Jagim, A 2024, 'Can Taking a Cold Plunge after Your Workout Be Beneficial?', *Mayo Clinic Health System,* viewed 25 February 2024, https://www.mayoclinichealthsystem.org/hometown-health/speaking-of-health/cold-plunge-after-workouts.

11   Ortega, MA, Fraile-Martinez, O, García-Montero, C, Callejón-Peláez, E, Sáez, MA, Álvarez-Mon, MA, García-Honduvilla, N, Monserrat, J, Álvarez-Mon, M, Bujan, J, & Canals, ML 2021, 'A General Overview on the Hyperbaric Oxygen Therapy: Applications, Mechanisms and Translational Opportunities', *Medicina (Kaunas, Lithuania)*, vol 57, no 9, p 864, viewed 14 April 2024, doi.org/10.3390/medicina57090864.

12   Oschman, JL, Chevalier, G, & Brown, R 2015, 'The Effects of Grounding (Earthing) on Inflammation, the Immune Response, Wound Healing, and Prevention and Treatment of Chronic Inflammatory and Autoimmune Diseases', *Journal of Inflammation Research*, vol 8, pp 83-96, viewed 14 April 2024, doi.org/10.2147/JIR.S69656.

13   Mahindru, A, Patil, P, & Agrawal, V 2023, 'Role of Physical Activity on Mental Health and Well-Being: A Review', *Cureus*, vol 15, no 1, viewed 25 February 2024, doi.org/10.7759/cureus.33475.

www.ingramcontent.com/pod-product-compliance
Lightning Source LLC
Chambersburg PA
CBHW022053020426
42335CB00012B/670